Dr. Scott's Knee Book

Symptoms, Diagnosis, and Treatment of Knee Problems,
Including: Torn Cartilage, Ligament Damage, Arthritis,
Tendinitis, Arthroscopic Surgery, and Total Knee Replacement

W. Norman Scott, M.D.

Chief, Division of Orthopaedics
Beth Israel Hospital, North Division, New York
Director, Insall Scott Kelly Institute for Orthopaedics
and Sports Medicine

and Carol Colman

Rehabilitative Strategies by Robert S. Gotlin, D.O.
Physician-in-charge
Beth Israel Hospital, North Division, New York
Orthopaedic Sports and Spine Rehabilitation

Illustrations by Johanna Warshaw

A FIRESIDE BOOK
Published by Simon & Schuster

New York   London   Toronto   Sydney   Tokyo   Singapore

FIRESIDE
Rockefeller Center
1230 Avenue of the Americas
New York, NY 10020

FIRESIDE and colophon are registered trademarks
of Simon & Schuster Inc.

Designed by Jeanette Olender
Manufactured in the United States of America

10   9   8

Library of Congress Cataloging-in-Publication Data
Scott, W. Norman.
[Knee book] Dr. Scott's knee book : symptoms, diagnosis, and
treatment of knee problems, including: torn cartilage, ligament damage, arthritis, tendinitis, arthroscopic surgery, and
total knee replacement / W. Norman Scott and Carol Colman ;
rehabilitative strategies by Robert S. Gotlin.
p. cm.   "A Fireside Book."
Includes index.
1. Knee—Wounds and injuries—Popular works.
2. Knee—Diseases—Popular works.
3. Knee—Surgery—Popular works.
I. Colman, Carol.   II. Gotlin, Robert S.   III. Title.
RD561.S396   1996   617.5'82—dc20
95-45405   CIP
ISBN 978-0-684-81104-8

CONTENTS

Introduction

If you're reading this book, you or someone you know probably has a knee problem. Maybe you've injured your knee while skiing or playing sports, or perhaps you're one of the millions of Americans who suffer from arthritis. You may have recently undergone knee surgery or are contemplating having surgery. Whatever the nature of your problem, you're not alone.

According to the American Academy of Orthopaedic Surgeons, some 4.2 million initial visits to doctors were made for knee problems in 1992 (the latest statistics available). That same year, another 1.3 million initial visits were made to emergency rooms because of knee injuries or knee pain. This is not surprising given the fact that nearly half of all people between 25 and 75 years old have experienced knee pain.

Many of them end up in my office. I am an orthopedic surgeon who specializes in the diagnosis and treatment of knee problems. At the Insall Scott Kelly Institute for Orthopaedics and Sports Medicine, affiliated with Beth Israel Medical Center in New York, I treat hundreds of patients each year for a wide variety of knee complaints. Knee problems don't discriminate. In my capacity as team doctor for the New York Knicks and former physician for the New York Rangers, my patients include some of the best-conditioned, finest athletes in the world. But I spend the majority of my time treating the so-called weekend athletes—people who sit at their desks all week long and, come Saturday or Sunday, play hard and sometimes get hurt. I also see a fair number of sedentary people who are not the slightest bit athletic and who have problem knees for different reasons.

Why are knee injuries so common? In order to answer this question, I need to explain a bit about the anatomy of the knee joint. By definition, a joint is a point in the body where two or more bones connect. In the case of the knee, however, the story is far more complex. The thigh bone (femur) connects to two bones: the shinbone (tibia), which lies directly underneath, and the fibula, a long bone on the outside of the leg. Another small bone, called the patella, or kneecap, sits on top between the two. Bones are connected to other bones by ligaments, thick fibrous bands of tissue. Muscles, which move the bones, are connected to them by tendons. The entire bone ends are lined in a smooth material called articular cartilage, which prevents the bones from rubbing against each other and allows them to glide smoothly. (For a full explanation of the parts of the knee, see Chapter 1.)

You may think that the knee is merely a hinge that connects the upper leg to the lower leg, but it is far more than that. The knee is actually an exquisitely designed machine. With every step you take, your knee is providing both stability and mobility. Your knee is designed to allow for a full range of motion— it moves from front to back, side to side, and up and down. It enables you to walk on a level surface, run up stairs, pivot, twist, and turn. You can kick your leg forward or fling it backward. You can stand, dance, swim, ski, or bicycle, thanks to your knees.

Your knees work very hard. The average person takes between 12,000 and 15,000 steps per day. With each step, your knees sustain a force of anywhere between two and seven times your body weight, depending on what you're doing. If you spend your day walking on carpet, the forces exerted through the knee are lower than if you're walking on hard pavement. If you jog or run, walk up stairs, or use a stair machine, the forces exerted through your knee can exceed 2,000 pounds! Over time, if your knee is continually bombarded and overworked, it will begin to "complain."

I don't mean to suggest that knee injuries are inevitable—far from it. One of the reasons I am writing this book is to show how many knee injuries can be prevented, and a good portion of this book is devoted to prevention. A good muscle-strengthening program is the best defense against knee injuries, and on page 160, I show you exactly what you need to do to protect against knee injuries. In addition, many people inadvertently do things that put their knees in jeopardy. Throughout this book, I offer advice on how to avoid activities that are true "knee killers." This book is also designed to help people whose knees are already "killing" them and are in the midst of considering their treatment options.

I am also writing this book because I feel that today, more than at any other time in our modern history, patients need to be fully informed. The cost-cutting environment in which medicine is being practiced is, in my opinion, detrimental to patient care. Physicians are often rushed and burdened with paperwork. Many insurance companies are so zealous to cut costs that they are actually discouraging patients from seeking appropriate care and refuse to pay for it when they do. Many patients in health maintenance organizations are finding it increasingly difficult to see a specialist of any kind, and knee surgeons are no exception.

As good as a general practitioner or internist may be, he or she cannot have the breadth of knowledge required to treat knee problems. The typical generalist has had at most a three-week rotation in all of orthopedic medicine as part of his or her medical training. The practice of orthopedics today, however, is highly technical and highly specialized. A physician who is not performing knee surgery and who is not up on the current literature is not going to be adept at making a diagnosis or designing a treatment plan. More and more, it is incumbent upon patients to arm themselves with the right information so that they can advocate for themselves. If present trends continue, only the most-educated, aggressive patients will be able to navigate through the health care system and get the care they need. This book is filled with important information that will help patients better find their way through the medical maze.

This book is also filled with good news. In recent years, there have been spectacular changes in the practice of orthopedic medicine that have revolutionized the diagnosis and treatment of knee problems. Knee surgery no longer means weeks or months of immobilization and a lengthy recovery period. More and more, surgery is being performed on an outpatient basis, and most people can walk out of the hospital with nothing more than an Ace bandage on their knee. A procedure called *arthroscopy* makes it possible for surgeons to perform intricate surgery through an incision about the size of a buttonhole. In many cases, a patient may come in for surgery in the morning, be up and around by afternoon, and go back to work the next day. A remarkable prosthesis—the total knee replacement—enables people who were once crippled with arthritis to enjoy pain-free mobility. Today, hundreds of thousands of Americans have total knee replacements, and many are not only walking, but are playing doubles tennis and even engaging in other sports.

In addition, there have been advancements made in the nonsurgical treatment of knee problems that are equally impressive, notably in the field of exercise rehabilitation. Under the direction of Robert Gotlin, D.O., the rehabilitation center at the Beth Israel Hospital, North Division, has made enormous strides in the treatment of knee problems. With the right exercise program, knee patients are able to regain motion and strength faster than ever before. With Dr. Gotlin's help, I have included several rehabilitation programs for common knee problems in this book.

Finally, I have written this book to dispel many of the myths that are commonly held about knee ailments. I have found that very often patients worry needlessly about the wrong things and ignore the really important ones. For example, patients are often very preoccupied with knee noise; they think that every creaking and cracking sound is an indication of a serious problem. It is not—noise without pain and swelling is not significant. But I can't tell you how many patients are certain that they have a "bum knee" because they hear these sounds. Pain is another symptom that is often misunderstood. People usually assume that pain is a sign of a serious problem. Paradoxically, when it comes to the knee, there is often no correlation between pain and degree of injury. A relatively healthy knee can hurt constantly, and yet a seriously "sick" knee may cause very little discomfort. Although this concept is difficult for patients to grasp (especially if they are the ones feeling the pain), once they become acquainted with the unique anatomy of the knee, which I explain in the next chapter, they will understand why pain is not the best way to diagnose a knee problem. They will also learn how to better manage their pain and, hopefully, reduce their discomfort to a minimum.

This book is not intended to replace your physician. Rather, the goal of this book is to help you work better with your physician. A knowledgeable patient will ask the right questions and will have realistic expectations about what to expect from each potential treatment. In the end, a well-informed patient will be able to make the right treatment choices and will be better prepared to work with his or her physician in a constructive way.

CHAPTER 1

Your Knee and How It Works

The knee joint consists of many different components which must work in sync to provide maximum stability and mobility. In this chapter, I describe the different parts of the knee, what they do, and how they work together.

The Fascia

Fascia is a strong, fibrous structure that encases the leg, providing protection and support. A taut layer of fascia can hold fat deposits under the skin in place, helping the knee to maintain a sleek appearance. As we age, however, fascia can lose some of its tone, which result in bulges of fatty tissue that can be mistaken for swelling. Due to the fact that women tend to be thinner than men, the bulging may be more noticeable in women.

Muscle

There are two groups of muscles that control the knee joint; the quadriceps and the hamstrings. Strong muscles are essential to protect and cushion bones and soft tissue (such as liga-

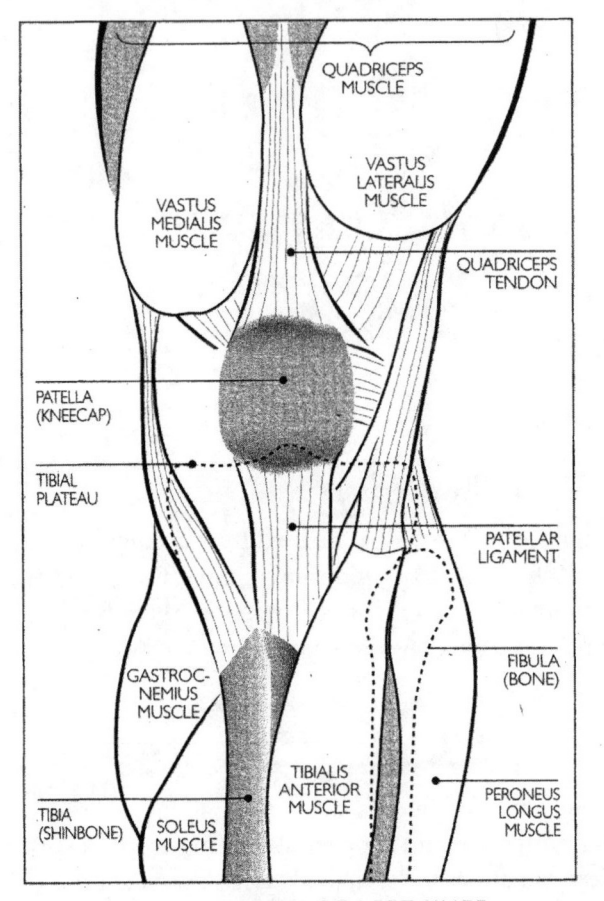

FRONTAL VIEW OF LEFT KNEE

ments and tendons) by absorbing the enormous forces that run through the knee.

The *quadriceps* are a collection of four muscles on the front of the thigh. Along with the quadriceps tendon, the patella (kneecap), and the patellar ligament, the quadriceps are responsible for the *extensor mechanism* of the leg, that is, the ability to straighten the knee or bring the bent knee to a straight position.

The *hamstring muscles*, on the back of the thigh, come

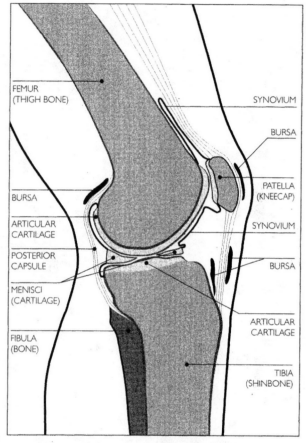

SIDE (MEDIAL) VIEW OF KNEE

down from the hip and the pelvis and insert below the knee. They control the knee by allowing it to go from an extended or straight position to a bent position.

The Capsule

The capsule is also a thick, fibrous type structure that wraps around the knee joint. Inside the capsule is soft tissue called

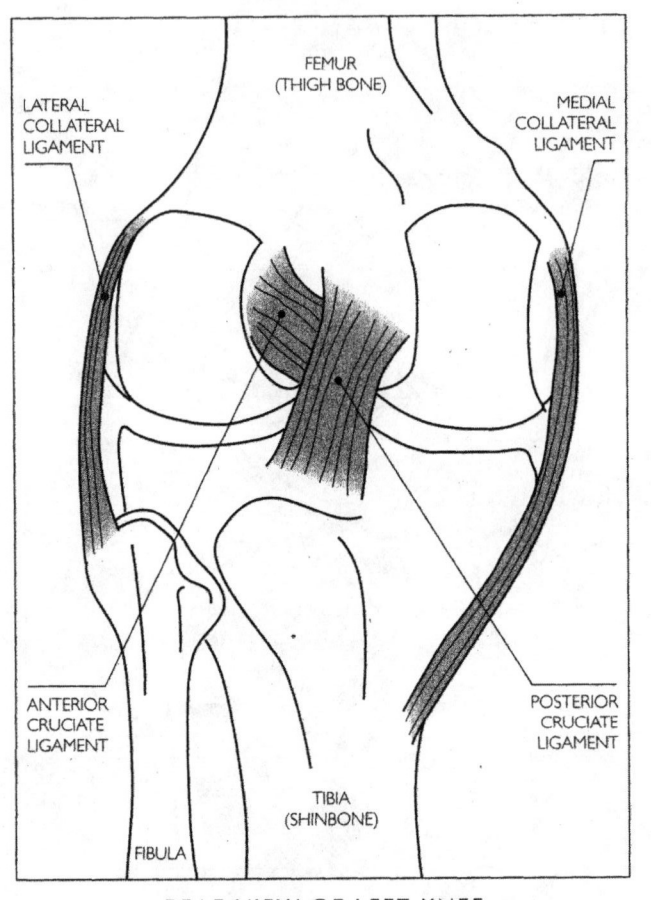

REAR VIEW OF LEFT KNEE

synovium. If the knee is injured, the synovium can become inflamed and will secrete excess synovial fluid as a protective mechanism. Inflammatory arthritis, such as rheumatoid arthritis, affects the synovium, which hypertrophies (thickens), secretes fluid, and can potentially destroy the articular cartilage and bone.

Bone

Bones provide strength, stability, and flexibility. They are shaped in such a way to allow you to flex and extend. There are four bones around the knee.

The *femur*, also known as the thigh bone, is the longest, largest, and strongest bone in the body. The femur runs down from the pelvis to the knee joint, where it meets with the tibia. The round knobs at the end of the bone are called *condyles*.

The *tibia*, also known as the shinbone, runs from the knee down to the ankle.

The *fibula* is a long, thin bone that begins below the knee and runs down the side of the leg (adjacent to the tibia) and ends at the ankles by forming a bulbous end called the *lateral malleolus,* the round knobs on the outside of your ankle. It is smaller and thinner than the tibia or femur.

The *patella*, also called the kneecap, is a small, flat triangular-shaped bone about 2 to 3 inches wide and 3 to 4 inches long that moves and rotates with the knee. The patella moves as the leg moves—it glides up and down the thigh bone almost as if it's on a track. Although it is small, the patella is a critical player in the mechanics of the knee. The patella is very important for muscle strength by giving the muscles the extra leverage they need to straighten the leg. The patella also cushions and protects the other bones of the joint. For example, in the case of a fall or blow to the knee, the patella may prevent the condyles (bony knobs) of the tibia or femur from being injured. If the patella slides off track even by a tiny amount, it can cause great pain and may result in permanent injury. If the kneecap partially comes off its track, it's called a *subluxation.* If the kneecap is entirely off track—for example, it sits way off to the side instead of in the center—it's called a *dislocation.*

Cartilage

The basic function of cartilage is to absorb shock and protect the bones. There are two types of cartilage in the knee joint: articular cartilage and the menisci.

The articular cartilage, also known as hyaline cartilage, is a white elastic material that lines the three bones that form the knee joint: the patella, femur and tibia. It is anywhere from 1/8 to 1/2 inch in thickness. Articular cartilage allows the knee (and other joints) to move in a fluid motion. Articular cartilage is composed primarily of water, collagen, and substances called *proteoglycans,* which are made up of large proteins and sugars. The wearing away of the articular cartilage, either through a traumatic injury or overuse, can result in arthritis. Softening or wearing away of the articular cartilage is called *chondromalacia.* Severe arthritis becomes evident when the hyaline cartilage is completely worn exposing raw bone (the subchondral bone).

Each knee has two *menisci:* the medial mensicus and lateral meniscus. (*Medial* refers to a part that is closest to the other leg, *lateral* refers to a part that is further away from the other leg.) The menisci are made of fibrous cartilage, a thick rubbery-type substance. Located on top of the tibial plateau, both menisci are basically shock absorbers, helping the knee withstand the enormous shear (side) forces that are placed on it daily. Meniscal injuries are fairly common, especially among athletes and are often a result of excessive force. Wear and tear due to age can also cause damage to the menisci.

Ligaments

Ligaments are strong, tough bands of white fibrous connective tissue, which link bones to bones. In the knee, ligaments primarily provide strength and stability from front to back, side to side, and rotational. There are several ligaments in the knee, however, the most important ones are the medial collateral ligament, the lateral collateral ligament, the anterior cruciate ligament, and the posterior cruciate ligaments.

The *medial collateral ligament* (MCL) runs down the inside of your knee joint, connecting the femur to the tibia and limiting the sideways motion of your knee. There are two parts: the superficial, which is longer, stronger, and more important, and the deep MCL. The MCL is vulnerable to a blow from the side, typical of contact sports such as football. If this ligament is injured, the knee may feel weak and wobbly.

The *lateral collateral ligament* (sometimes called the fibula collateral ligament) runs on the outside of your knee from the femur to the fibula and limits sideways motion.

The *anterior cruciate ligament* (ACL), located deep in your knee, connects the femur to the tibia in the center of your knee, limiting rotation and the forward motion of the tibia. The ACL is especially vulnerable to injury caused by a sudden twisting motion.

The *posterior cruciate ligament* (PCL), also located deep in the knee, connects the femur to the tibia, limiting the backward motion of the knee. The PCL is the strongest ligament and is usually injured with more extreme force, such as a car accident.

Tendons

There are two major tendons about the knee: the quadriceps tendon and the patellar tendon.

By definition, a tendon connects muscle to bone. However, the *patellar tendon* connects the patella (kneecap) to the tibia (shinbone), which means that the patellar tendon is really a ligament. Through the years, this ligament has become known colloquially as a tendon, and to prevent confusion, I will call it the patellar tendon throughout this book.

The quadriceps tendon connects the quadriceps muscle to the patella and thus provides power for leg extension.

Overuse of any tendon can result in tendinitis, which may cause local pain and tenderness.

Plicae

Plicae are embryological remnants of synovial folds—basically a dividing line along the joint in the embryo. As the embryo matures, the dividing lines are no longer needed, and they often rupture spontaneously. However, these long, elastic plicae (similar to rubber bands) remain in about 70 percent of all people. Plicae rarely cause problems; however, in some cases, the bands or folds can get caught between the femur and kneecap and can cause pain.

In the chapters to come, you will see how all of these components must work together to keep your knee strong and well functioning and what can happen when things go awry. In the next chapter, I will discuss what every patient needs to know to get an accurate diagnosis for a knee problem.

CHAPTER 2

Getting to a Correct Diagnosis

A thorough examination by a skilled and experienced physician is a critical first step in diagnosing knee problems. In fact, if properly done, the physical examination can result in a diagnosis of anywhere between 80 and 90 percent accuracy. If necessary, further testing can achieve an accuracy rate of nearly 100 percent. This chapter will not only review state of the art diagnostic techniques, but will show patients how they can work with their physicians to help achieve an accurate diagnosis.

Before the physician begins the physical examination, he or she will take a thorough medical history of the patient. Therefore, you should be prepared to provide your physician with relevant information that could help determine your diagnosis.

Family Medical History

Some orthopedic problems may be hereditary. Be sure to tell your physician about any significant family illnesses that might shed some light on your problem. These include a primary relative (e.g., sibling, parent, or grandparent) with a condition such as arthritis or gout or a relative with a congenital abnormality such as a dislocated kneecap. Obviously, your physician need not know about nonhereditary orthopedic problems.

Personal Medical History

Inform your physician about any past injuries or significant illnesses. Be sure to tell your physician if you were ever on steroids for a medical problem, even if it was for a short time. People who took steroids—even low doses for short periods of time—are more prone to develop avascular necrosis, a condition characterized by poor blood supply to the knee joint. Although the exact cause of the condition is unknown, it appears as if the small vessels that feed the joint become blocked, resulting in inadequate blood supply to the knee joint. The cartilage in the joint eventually dies and collapses, which can lead to severe arthritis. In addition, people with a history of alcoholism are also at risk of developing avascular necrosis.

If you have had a history of knee problems, tell your doctor, even if the problem was a seemingly minor one. A past sprain—even if it occurred several decades ago—could prove to be significant today. It helps to describe your problems as simply as possible, since patients may use medical terms inaccurately, and this can lead to confusion. For example, patients often say that their knees "lock." When questioned further, they may explain, "Well, my knee goes into spasm," or "My knee hurts when I move it." The true definition of locking, however, is the inability to extend the knee. Therefore, avoid using labels when describing any past (or present) problems and just tell your doctor how you feel. It's the best history.

If you have recently been sick—if you've had a high fever, are experiencing pain in other joints, are excessively fatigued, or had any other unusual symptoms—alert your doctor. Several diseases, including Lyme disease, systemic lupus erythematosus, and rheumatoid arthritis, could present with all or some of these symptoms. In addition to causing knee problems, they can progressively worsen unless properly treated. Strep infection (strep throat), caused by the streptococcus bacteria, could also cause temporary arthritic symptoms. If your doctor suspects that your knee problem may actually be caused by one of these diseases, he will order special diagnostic blood tests and often aspirate fluid from the knee.

Symptoms

As a rule, orthopedists see two types of patients: first, patients who have recently suffered from an acute injury and are seeking immediate medical attention, and second, patients with chronic problems. These patients have often been in discomfort for some time and have learned to live with it. They seek help only when their symptoms take a turn for the worse.

The acute patient should be able to give a fairly accurate account of how the injury happened. If possible, write down a brief description of the injury while it is still fresh in your mind. It can be very helpful to a physician to hear details such as "I was playing tennis, I reached for a backhand, and I twisted my foot. Then I heard a pop. Suddenly, I was in tremendous pain and I couldn't continue playing." Based on this description, a physician might suspect a ligament problem, which could be verified by further testing.

It is also helpful if patients can help localize the pain. I often ask patients to—without stopping to think—quickly point to the exact spot where it hurts. By isolating the precise location of pain, it may further narrow down the possible diagnosis.

The chronic patient may not be able to pinpoint the exact time when the problem began, but you, too, can provide invaluable information. Most importantly, you should be able to tell the doctor when and where your knee bothers you, and what activities seem to make it better or worse. Be as specific as possible; keep a diary if need be. Does your knee bother you when you walk or when you run? Does it hurt when you walk up stairs? Does it hurt when you get up from a chair? Does it hurt more at night than during the day? Is the knee swollen, or does it swell after certain activities? The answers to these questions may offer important clues as to what your problem is.

It is also important for the chronic patient to tell the doctor about the degree to which you rely on pain medication such as aspirin, ibuprofen, or any other anti-inflammatory drug, either prescription or over the counter. If you can't make it through the day without a hefty dose of painkillers, your doctor should know about it. It is also important to identify when you may need to take medication. For example, if you're pain free except when you're playing tennis, or dancing, it could provide some clues as to the cause of your problem.

The Physical Examination

After taking a thorough patient history, your physician will begin the physical examination. The examination is based on inspection, what your physician can actually see, and palpation, what your physician can touch and feel.

Alignment

Alignment very simply refers to how your bones—from your hip, to your knee, all the way down to your foot and ankle—stack up in relation to each other. The bones must be aligned in such a way that allows for both stability and flexibility. A minor variation in alignment is not serious; however, if the alignment is truly out of whack, it could cause pain and serious problems.

What's normal alignment? Theoretically, the patella (kneecap) should rest in the center of the knee, and the tibia

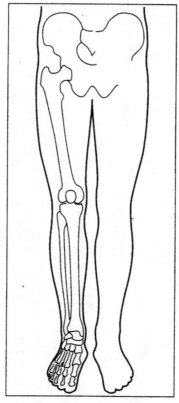

NORMAL ALIGNMENT

(shinbone) should stand directly underneath. A perfectly straight knee joint is designated at 0 degrees, meaning neither side of the body is favored. However, in reality, more people have knees that are aligned slightly out or in. In fact, women are normally slightly knock-kneed, meaning their knees appear as if they rotate in toward each other. In order to maintain balance, their tibias are slightly angled outward away from the midline of the body at about 5 to 7 degrees. When the tibia points away from the midline, it is called *valgus* alignment. Men tend to have less valgus knee joints. In fact, more men than women are bowlegged, meaning their knees appear

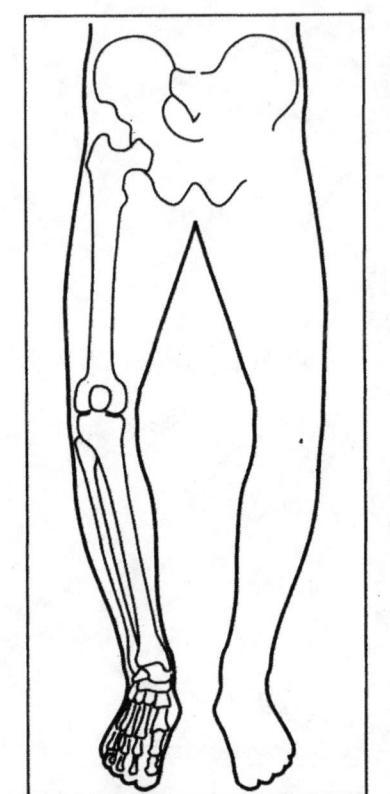 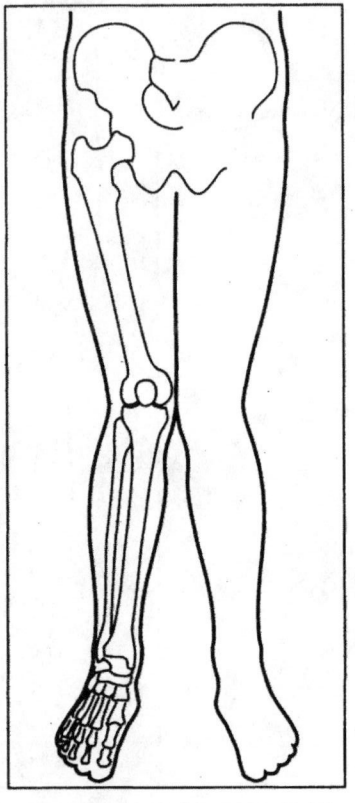

BOWLEGGED (VARUS)   KNOCK-KNEED (VALGUS)
ALIGNMENT   ALIGNMENT

to go out while their tibias curve in toward the midline of the body. When the tibia points toward the midline, it is called *varus* alignment.

Alignment irregularities can sometimes point to a particular problem. For example, knock-kneed deformities are more common in rheumatoid arthritis, and bowlegged deformities are more common in osteoarthritis, the kind of wear and tear arthritis associated with old age.

Abrasions

Your physician will examine the knee for any signs of puncture wounds or abrasions. A small cut that could easily go unnoticed by the patient could have become infected, causing pain and inflammation.

Swelling

The knee joint is normally filled with a tiny amount of fluid for lubrication. However, when the joint is injured, the synovium (the soft tissue inside the knee capsule) responds by producing even more fluid to protect the joint—the so-called synovial response. A synovial response is usually delayed because the synovium has to produce the synovial fluid. Swelling due to the synovial response is typical of a meniscal injury not related to the meniscal blood supply.

Swelling may also be due to a rupture of a blood vessel, which causes immediate bleeding and results in immediate swelling within an hour after the injury. This is more typical of a ligament injury, fracture, or dislocated kneecap.

Many older patients may think that their knees are swollen all the time, but this may not be the case. Very often, as we age, the fascia, which encases the leg, may lose some of its tautness, resulting in bulges of fatty tissue. How do you test for true swelling? If you straighten out both of your legs to about kneecap level, you should see a small indentation or dimple on the medial side. In the case of real swelling, the dimple will look more like a pouch.

There are other reasons that a knee may look swollen but isn't. For example, arthritic knees may appear to be enlarged due to bone spurs or osteophytes, which are bone growths that develop as a result of the erosion of cartilage. The loss of cartilage may cause instability, and the formation of osteophytes can help to stabilize the joint, probably by increasing the surface area.

Point of Tenderness

Your physician will feel around the knee to determine precisely where it hurts. Does it hurt in the area of the kneecap? Does it hurt in the area of the meniscus? Although it may not be possible to pinpoint the precise trouble spot, this examination can give your doctor some idea of where the problem may lie.

Sometimes the pain may be isolated to one spot; sometimes it may seem to roam all over the knee. When the physician says, "Where does it hurt?" in about 20 percent of all cases, a patient with kneecap symptoms will specifically point to the patella. However, 20 percent will point to the left side of the knee, 20 percent will point to the right side, 20 percent will complain of pain in the back of the knee, and 20 percent will say that they have pain everywhere. This is not surprising: pain is often referred, that is, an injury in one location may hurt in another. In the case of the knee joint, the closeness of the anatomy makes it even more difficult to precisely pinpoint the location of the pain, but an experienced specialist can often narrow down the possibilities.

Range of Motion

Your physician will move your leg in various ways to check the range of motion, the ability to straighten and bend the knee. A healthy knee should be able to bend and flex with ease. Pain or restricted movement could suggest several possible problems. For example, perhaps the patella is not aligned correctly. Or if there is pain upon compressing the joint (when you flex or bend your foot toward your back), it means that there are ar-

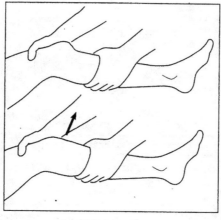

LACHMAN TEST

ticular cartilage problems. If the leg gets "locked" upon extension or straightening, it might suggest a displaced meniscal tear or a subluxed (offtrack) patella.

Tests for Stability

Ligaments are strong bands of connective tissue that connect bones to bones and provide strength and stability. Ligaments give the knee the necessary flexibility to move in different directions without throwing the leg off balance. If a ligament is injured—if it is stretched out or torn—it will allow for excessive movement, which may make the leg feel wobbly. There are several tests for stability that may help your physician determine which, if any, ligaments may be injured. In each of these tests, your physician will move each leg in such a way that stresses a particular ligament and will compare one leg in relation to the other. She will straighten, bend, flex, and rotate the leg. If the leg has too much slack—for example, if it "gives" too much in either direction—or if the patient feels pain, it suggests that that particular ligament is injured.

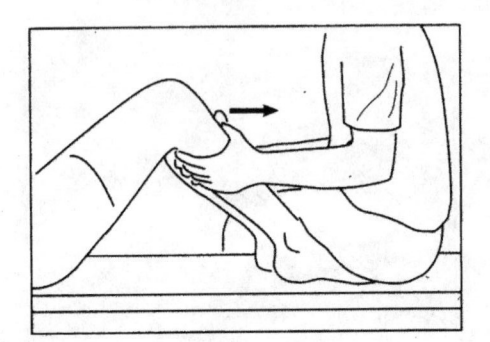

ANTERIOR DRAWER TEST

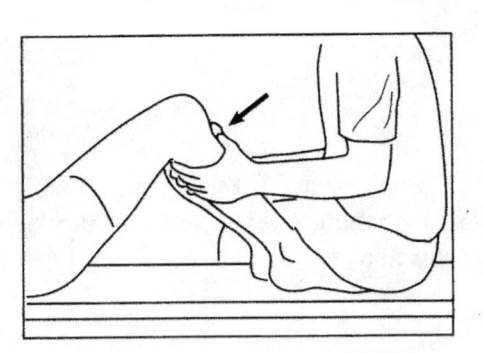

POSTERIOR DRAWER TEST

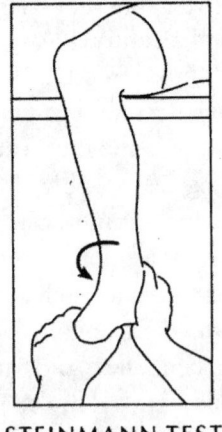

STEINMANN TEST

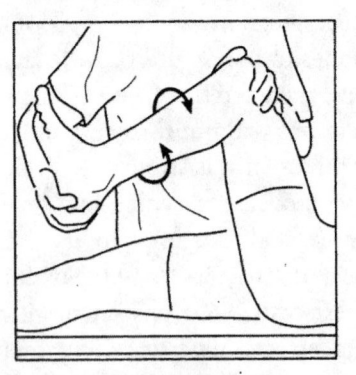

McMURRAY TEST

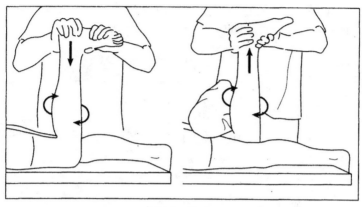

APLEY TEST

Ligament injuries are called sprains and are classified according to degree of severity ranging from grade 1, the most benign, to grade 3, the most serious. In a grade 1 sprain, the knee does not move excessively, which means the ligament is still intact; however, the patient may be in pain. In a grade 2 sprain, the knee will open up less than 5 millimeters. In a grade 3 sprain, the ligament will open all the way to 1 centimeter, and the knee is wobbly.

There are several tests that are commonly used to diagnose specific ligament problems.

Medial Collateral Ligament (MCL)

The MCL prevents the leg from turning to the outside. To test the stability of this ligament, your physician will apply a force to the outside of the leg and gently tug. If the MCL is intact, the knee will not move. However, if it's torn or damaged, the knee will feel painful, or it will swing out too far.

Lateral Collateral Ligament (LCL)

The LCL prevents the leg from turning inside toward the other leg. To test the stability of this ligament, your doctor will apply force on the inside of your leg and pull it toward the other leg. If you feel pain or the leg rotates too much toward the other leg, it is a sign that the LCL may be injured.

Anterior Cruciate Ligament (ACL)

The ACL limits rotation and forward motion of the tibia. The Lachman test is often used to test the ACL. In this test, your doctor will put your leg in 10 to 15 degrees of flexion and then pull forward on the tibia, almost as if she's trying to pull the tibia away. If the knee moves 3 to 5 millimeters or more from the other knee, it could signify a torn ACL.

Posterior Cruciate Ligament (PCL)

The PCL limits the backward motion of the knee. The posterior draw test is used to test the PCL. In this test, your doctor will bend your knee 90 degrees and push the tibia back. If it moves more than 5 millimeters, it's a sign of a torn PCL.

In the right hands, stability tests can be very accurate. However, they must be done by an experienced practitioner who is able to discern subtle movements in the leg—so minute they can be measured in millimeters—and equally subtle differences between legs that may be clinically significant.

Meniscal Injuries

Each knee contains two menisci made of fibrous cartilage, which are basically shock absorbers. The Steinmann test is one of the tests used to diagnose meniscal injuries. In this test, your physician will have you sit up on a table with your legs hanging over the side. Your physician will then twist each leg, moving it in and out. If you feel pain in the meniscal area, it may indicate a meniscal problem.

The Apley and McMurray tests can also be helpful in diagnosing a meniscal tear. In the Apley test, you are prone, knee bent 90 degrees, and the foot rotated inward and outward. This compressive and rotational force will often signal a medial or lateral meniscal tear. In the McMurray test, you are supine, the knee bent fully (approximately 130 to 140 degrees) and slowly extended while externally rotated. A loud pop might signify a torn medial meniscus. Unfortunately, however, there are often lots of noises in a knee that are harmless, and such an event while performing a McMurray test might be misleading to the inexperienced physician.

Laboratory Tests

X Ray

Every knee patient should have an X ray, a photographic image of inside the body. X rays are important for several reasons. First, they help to rule out other conditions such as tumors or fractures. In fact, there are several reported cases of people being treated for knee problems who in reality had tumors that went undiagnosed because they had never been X rayed. Second, because X rays provide a good view of large bones, they are excellent for diagnosing alignment problems and detailing later stages of arthritis. If the joint spaces are abnormally small, that is, if the bones are too close together, it's a good indication that the articular cartilage is worn away and the patient is arthritic.

In order for an X ray to be useful, however, it must be taken correctly, and that's easier said than done. Many of the X rays I see are incomplete, especially those that are taken in an emergency room. Very often, they show only one or at most two views of the knee, and that simply does not offer enough information to make an intelligent diagnosis. A good set of knee X rays should include several views of the knee in various positions, extended and flexed, from the front, side, and back. In addition, in the case of an older person who might be arthritic, the X ray should be taken standing up. If the patient is sitting or lying down, the joint spaces could look normal, and only when the person is standing will the joint spaces narrow.

If you are getting an X ray and the technician only takes one or two views, I think it's a sign that something is not being done correctly. In many cases—especially if the X ray is being done in a hectic emergency room—the technician may be cutting corners or he simply may not know the right way to X ray a knee. Don't be afraid to speak up. Ask to see an orthopedist, or at the very least say, "If you're concerned enough to order an X ray of my knee, I want it read by a radiologist or an orthopedist." In reality, the orthopedist is quite often more informed than a radiologist who does not have a primary interest in orthopedic radiology.

X rays are good for looking at bones, but they are unable to provide a good view of soft tissue, such as ligaments and muscles. If your doctor feels that your problem is not bone related and she is unable to diagnose it with a thorough physical examination, she may order additional tests.

Computerized Axial Tomographic Scanning (CAT scan)

A CAT scan is a tubelike X ray that attempts to define the three-dimensional aspects of the bone. At one time, these machines were loud, clumsy, and uncomfortable, with the patient slowly moving through a long tube. With the new technologies, these machines are quieter and more comfortable, with the patient simply lying on the examining table as the scanner passes over him.

A regular X ray provides a two-dimensional view of bone; a CAT scan can view slices of bone section by section. By piecing together these sections, the surgeon can get a three-dimensional view of the problem. A CAT scan is useful as a surgical tool in cases of bone cancer because it enables the surgeon to see the extent of the tumor embedded within the bone. Tibial plateau or distal femoral fractures are often scanned to better assess the three-dimensional nature of these injuries.

Bone Scan

In a bone scan, a radioactive material is injected into the bloodstream and the patient is placed on a board in a scanner—a long narrow tube—and must lie still for about 30 minutes as the scanner "picks up" the radioactive material at the appropriate sites. Some of the newer scanning machines are open and slowly move over the patient. As the radioactive material travels through the blood, the physician can scan the phases of the blood flow. From this test, the physician can see how the blood pools in any particular area as contrasted to normal values. Changes in the normal values may be indicative of infection, avascular necrosis, or some bone tumors.

Magnetic Resonance Imaging (MRI)

If a doctor suspects a patient has a ligament problem or a torn meniscus, she may order an MRI to confirm the diagnosis. The MRI is also good at identifying bone bruises—abrasions on the bone that may have been caused by an injury and could cause pain. MRI uses a strong magnetic field and radio waves to look inside the body and create images that are analyzed by a computer. For the MRI, the patient is put on a table and told to lie still. The patient is then slowly moved through a long tube in which different views of the knee are recorded. Some MRI machines are totally enclosed; some are just partially enclosed.

Similar to an X ray, an MRI cannot image articular cartilage. However, as the computer software becomes more technologically sophisticated, I suspect that it probably will be able to diagnose articular cartilage problems in the future.

The MRI is only as good as its human operators, and the results that I see are often inadequate. A complete MRI of the knee should take about 45 minutes, allowing for views of the knee from every 2 to 3 millimeters at many different angles. Many of the films I see are of poor quality, I suspect because the test was rushed either for cost containment or because the technician didn't know any better. It's a waste of your time and money. Therefore, I recommend that you only go to an MRI center that has been recommended by an orthopedist.

An MRI costs about $1,000 and offers a degree of accuracy ranging from as low as 60 percent to a high of 90 percent for ligament and meniscal tears. A good clinical exam by an experienced physician can offer almost the same degree of accuracy. Therefore, there is some controversy as to whether an MRI is really that useful and cost-effective. However, in this age of "second opinions," many insurance companies require an MRI before surgery.

Another problem with the MRI is interpretation. The radiologist rarely, if ever, compares MRI films to arthroscopic findings; thus, the orthopedist usually has more constant feedback and subsequently a better ability to interpret the MRI.

In some cases, the MRI may reveal nothing, and if the patient is in pain, the physician may order additional tests.

Arthroscopy

Arthroscopy (also called a "scope") of the knee is a surgical procedure that has revolutionized the way that knee problems are both diagnosed and treated. Prior to the arthroscope, open knee surgery (arthrotomies)—actually making an incision in the knee that is several inches long—was the only way to get a complete view of the knee joint. The procedure (which is still used for certain operations such as total knee replacement, patella realignment, and fracture treatment) requires hospitalization and usually a longer recovery period than the scope. Arthroscopy has eliminated the need for open-knee surgery for many patients. Thanks to fiberoptic technology, it is now possible to look inside the knee through an incision roughly the size of a small buttonhole.

Arthroscopy is performed in a hospital operating room or an outpatient surgical suite. During an arthroscopic procedure, the patient is first anesthetized either by general or local anesthetic. Although the procedure can be performed under a local, I rarely use local anesthesia without intravenous sedatives. Local injections can be painful, but a "twilight" sleep can eliminate all discomfort. In addition, local anesthesia is often partially ineffective causing periods of intense pain during the surgical procedure, thus compromising the exam. An arthroscopy as a rule cannot be properly performed unless the patient is extremely cooperative and totally relaxed.

Once the patient is under the anesthesia, a sterile solution is injected into the joint to expand it. In most cases, the physician will use a tourniquet device around the thigh (similar to a blood pressure cuff) to prevent bleeding. (If only a local anesthetic is used, the tourniquet can be quite painful.) The physician then punctures two or three small incisions in the skin of the knee and inserts a pencil-shaped arthroscope, a miniature lens and light that greatly magnifies and illuminates the inside of the joint. Images from inside the joint are displayed on a nearby television screen. During the arthroscopy, the physician not only can look directly into the joint, but can palpate, or feel, the ligaments, menisci, and other relevant structures. (An MRI may show that a meniscus or ligament is torn, but only an arthroscope can verify whether the tear is a significant one.) If the meniscal or ligament tear is serious, the surgeon can repair it during the procedure using tiny pen-sized surgical instruments in the joint. Thus, the surgery can be performed with a minimum of trauma to the patient. In addition, unlike other diagnostic tests, arthroscopy provides a clear view of the articular cartilage and can delineate any damage.

In most cases, a combined diagnostic and therapeutic

arthroscopy lasts less than an hour, and the recovery from both a diagnostic and therapeutic scope is the same. After the arthroscopy is completed, the incisions are closed and bandaged. In fact, within an hour after the procedure, many patients are able to go home with nothing more than an Ace bandage on their knee. Each case is different: talk to your physician about what you can realistically expect in terms of pain and recovery time. Ice applied to the injured area and pain medication can help reduce swelling and discomfort.

Arthroscopy of the knee is best performed by a skilled practitioner who does the procedure routinely. In order to be truly adept at arthroscopy, a surgeon should have done at least two hundred and fifty to five hundred of these procedures. You don't want to be arthroscoped by a surgeon who only does a handful of arthroscopies each year. As good a surgeon as he/she may be, he/she may miss something that a more experienced surgeon would have observed. If performed by an experienced practitioner, arthroscopy is virtually 100 percent accurate for determining a diagnosis. However, arthroscopy is rarely done for purely diagnostic purposes. More often, a physician will suspect a particular problem, verify the diagnosis during arthroscopy, and then correct it at the same time.

Arthroscopy is a powerful diagnostic tool; however, it is not a panacea. Many patients with knee pain or discomfort may undergo arthroscopy with high hopes that it will cure their problem only to have their hopes dashed when the arthroscopy reveals that their problem stems from the destruction of articular cartilage for which there is no quick fix. These patients are understandably disappointed and often angry. To avoid this situation, I feel it's important for patients to understand the limitations of arthroscopy before undergoing the procedure. Be sure to ask your doctor what you stand to gain from this procedure and whether your particular problem is one that can actually be corrected.

Albeit rare, arthroscopy is not without risk. Because it is an invasive procedure, there is always the risk of infection, which occurs in less than 1 percent of all patients. There is also a small (less than 1 percent) risk of nerve damage, which could result in loss of ankle and foot function, and a handful of other potentially troublesome problems, such as reflex sympathetic dystrophy, a stiff, painful joint in which the cause is unknown and fortunately rarely occurs. Although complications potentially exist, I want to stress that the overwhelming number of arthroscopic procedures are both safe and successful.

Tests for Related Problems

If your physician suspects that your knee problem is being caused by an infection or other problem, she will order the following additional blood tests.

Complete Blood Count (CBC)

If your physician feels that a recent infection may have caused your knee problems, she will order a CBC. An excess of white blood cells may point to a bacterial infection. An inflamed, swollen joint may also be indicative of an inflammatory arthritis for which there is a specific blood test such as rheumatoid arthritis or systemic lupus erythematosus. These inflammatory joint problems are believed to be autoimmune in origin. (An autoimmune disease is characterized by a malfunction of the patient's own immune system in which the patient produces antibodies against his own tissue. The connective tissue—cartilage, tendons, and collagen—are particularly vulnerable.)

Rheumatoid Factor

If you are experiencing pain or discomfort in other joints or if you have a family history of rheumatoid arthritis, your physician may order a blood test for rheumatoid factor. About 75 percent of all patients with rheumatoid arthritis will test positive. If you have rheumatoid arthritis, your physician will refer you to a rheumatologist, a specialist in connective tissue disease, for treatment. The knee surgeon is consulted when the knee problems can no longer be managed with anti-inflammatory medication.

Systemic Lupus Erythematosus

Similar to rheumatoid arthritis, systemic lupus erythematosus is an autoimmune disease that primarily strikes women and can cause joint pain and arthritic-type symptoms such as stiffness and swelling. If you have a family history of lupus or any other symptoms that may point to this diagnosis, your physician will order several blood tests to screen for this disease. Basically, these tests all look for specific markers in the blood that are often found in lupus patients. If you have lupus, your physician will refer you to a rheumatologist for treatment.

Lyme Titer

Joint pain and inflammation can be symptoms of Lyme disease. If you live in the Northeast or in an area where Lyme is prevalent or if you've been in a tick-infested area, your physician may order a Lyme titer, a screening test for Lyme disease. Lyme disease is treated with antibiotics. Very often, the arthritic symptoms associated with Lyme will disappear after the patient recovers.

CHAPTER 3

What Can Go Wrong

Meniscal Injuries

I played football in college, now I'm an attorney and I'm on my feet all day arguing cases. Many nights, I go out dancing. I recently put on a lot of weight. I was born bowlegged. All of this took its toll on my knee. My knee started hurting, the pain would travel down to my ankles by night. I could barely stand up. My doctor said I had a torn meniscus and recommended that I have arthroscopic surgery to repair it. I didn't like the idea of surgery, but I felt if I wanted to get on with my life, I had no choice.

John, thirty-four years old

The menisci are made of fibrous cartilage, which is composed of collagen bundles. They are thick, rubbery structures that are attached to the tibia and the fibula. There are two menisci in each knee: the medial meniscus (on the inner side of the knee joint) and the lateral meniscus (on the outside of the knee). The menisci serve as a cushion or shock absorber, protecting the knee bones from excess force.

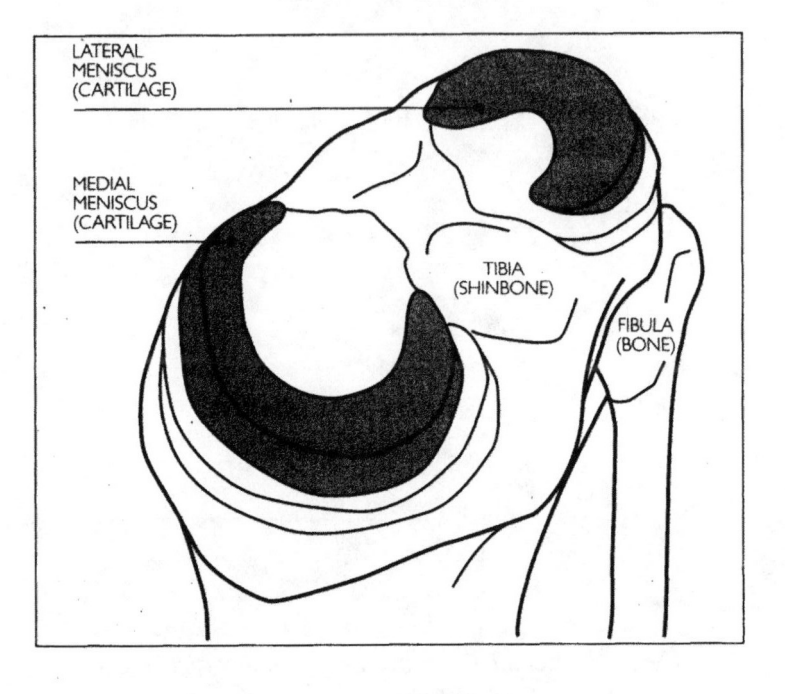

Both menisci are crescent-shaped discs; the medial meniscus is longer from front to back than the lateral meniscus,
which is shaped more like an open C. The lateral meniscus has
a looser connection to the capsule of the joint and, therefore,
has more mobility.

At one time, it was believed that the menisci had no particular function, and in fact, if they became injured or torn, then
one or both could be removed without inpunity. Today, orthopedists have a new appreciation for the menisci and the critical role they play as shock absorbers. We now believe that
people with damaged menisci may be more prone to develop
arthritis. In fact, meniscectomy (removal of a meniscus) is performed only as a last resort—we try very hard to repair and
preserve this important piece of cartilage.

Some people may have a congenital abnormality of the lateral meniscus called a *discoid meniscus*. Instead of the usual C
shape, the meniscus is flat and pancakelike. Before the days of

arthroscopy, doctors believed that a discoid meniscus was a major cause of pain and discomfort. In fact, a click of the knee was considered absolute evidence of a discoid meniscus, and the troublesome cartilage was typically removed. Unfortunately, the diagnosis was often wrong. (The knee can click for many different reasons, most of them harmless.) In addition, from the hindsight of observing thousands of patients during arthroscopy, we have learned that a discoid meniscus is not only benign, but because it covers more surface, it may actually be a better shock absorber. However, there is still some controversy as to whether a discoid meniscus tears more easily than a normal meniscus.

The menisci are particularly susceptible to injury due to the rotational forces that are placed on them. For example, when you walk or run, you're not just moving your knee forward or back, your knee also rotates slightly to allow for a pivoting motion. Your knee joint must move in sync to correctly absorb the forces that are placed on it. However, what may happen is when you move suddenly or make a quick, twisting motion, the femur may rotate, but the foot remains fixed. As a result, the joint is not allowed to go through its normal motion, and the meniscus can get caught in the middle and is torn either partially or completely apart. Although meniscal injuries can happen to anyone, athletes who perform sports that require running and pivoting are particularly prone to them. Not surprisingly, it's a frequent injury among basketball players. Torquing right and then pivoting left with a fixed foot—a typical basketball maneuver—is a common mechanism of meniscal injury.

But most meniscal injuries occur off the basketball court in the most mundane of situations. For example, a more typical scenario is one in which you're getting up from a chair or you trip off a curb, and suddenly you feel pain in your knee. The knee swells up later in the day or overnight, and it may feel more comfortable keeping the leg in a bent or flexed position. You limp around a bit and hope that the pain goes away, but it often persists and eventually you end up at the doctor's office. Your doctor will probably order a magnetic resonance image (MRI), and although the MRI will show a meniscal injury, it cannot pinpoint the precise date of the injury. (Only arthroscopy can distinguish between a new and chronic tear.) The meniscal injury that is causing you grief today could have been the result of a tear from years or even decades in the past. At the time, the injury may not have been serious and may have even gone unnoticed but nevertheless left the meniscus vulnerable to further injury. The rather insignificant event that triggered the pain (getting up from the chair or tripping off the curb) was the "final straw" that led to a more serious injury.

MRIs of people over fifty have revealed that the menisci appear to undergo a degenerative process due to aging. In older people, the menisci routinely soften: the collagen bundles loosen up much the same way collagen loosens up in skin, which causes aging skin to wrinkle. The once strong surface of the meniscus becomes filled with deposits of fat rather than tense, fibrous tissue. Although the aging meniscus may loose some of its strength, it still has some shock-absorbing function. We don't know exactly what percentage of the normal load-bearing forces a degenerative meniscus can withstand, but studies reveal that keeping a symptom-free meniscus is better than completely removing it, which will inevitably lead to arthritic changes.

In fact, on an MRI, a meniscus of an older person may appear to be far worse than it actually is and may not be the cause of the person's pain or discomfort.

Types of Meniscal Tears

There are various types of meniscal injuries ranging in severity and impact. Depending on the strength and type of force exerted on it, the meniscus can tear in any number of ways; it can split in half, it can get a so-called parrot beak tear (which

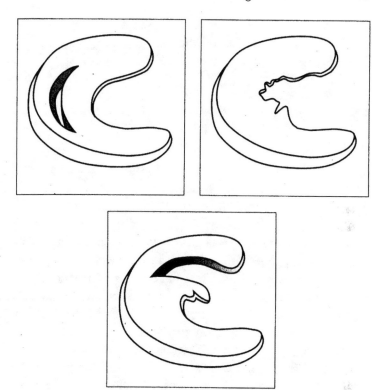

REPRESENTATIVE PATTERNS OF MENISCAL TEARS

is actually a cleavage or radial tear), or it can rip around its circumference in the shape of a C. The meniscus can withstand a tiny tear in which it retains its connection to the front and back of the knee joint or a major tear in which it is left hanging on by a thread. One of the most common tears is a bucket handle tear, a crescent-shaped tear in which the meniscus remains attached at the front and back of the remaining meniscus. The degree of seriousness for any tear depends on its location and what percentage of the meniscus is torn: a 10 percent tear is insignificant but a 50 percent tear is serious. In other words, the bigger the tear, the more troublesome it becomes.

In addition to causing pain and discomfort, a torn or displaced meniscus can abraid the articular cartilage, thus increasing the chances of getting arthritis.

Diagnosing Meniscal Problems

Patient History

An injured meniscus will typically result in tenderness and swelling at the joint line. However, in the case of an acute injury, an observant patient can further help clarify the diagnosis. To the trained ear, there is a big difference between a patient who reports, "I was playing tennis and then suddenly I was in so much pain that they had to carry me off the court and my knee swelled up like a balloon," and a patient who says, "I was playing tennis last night, and my knee hurt a little but I continued playing, but by morning, my knee was really swollen." The degree of pain and the timing of swelling can provide important diagnostic clues as to the location and severity of the injury. Here's why. The blood supply to the meniscus, which comes from the capsule, flows from the outer part of the meniscus to the middle. As a result, there is a very good supply of blood to the peripheral or outer part of the meniscus, called the red zone. However, as you move from the periphery to the middle of the meniscus, the blood supply becomes scarce—the so-called white zone. Nerve endings tend to follow the blood vessels. Pain is a reflection of the synovial reaction or inflammation throughout the joint. If there is a peripheral tear, blood will immediately spill into the joint. If no blood vessels are disrupted, the synovium will secrete fluid, a delayed response, which results in a collection of fluid several hours later.

The timing of swelling can also help to pinpoint the location of the injury. Immediate swelling means that blood vessels have been ruptured, a sign that the injury occurred in the red zone or is more typical of a ligament injury. Delayed swelling, swelling that begins 6 to 12 hours after an injury, is a sign that the joint has filled up with fluid as a result of inflammation, the so-called synovial response.

Physical Exam

In addition to palpating for pain and swelling, the physician will turn the knee in such a way that it stresses the meniscal attachment to the capsule. If the patient experiences pain, it is often localized to the site of the tear. Although it would seem straightforward to palpate the meniscus, it isn't. The structures are in such proximity that only an experienced knee surgeon can delineate the difference between the meniscus, articular cartilage, synovium, and capsule.

Your physician will also check for range of motion. A person with an injured meniscus may be unable to extend his leg comfortably and may feel better in a flexed position—in fact, in many cases, the knee will lock. At one time, it was believed that the meniscus somehow got caught in the joint and was obstructing movement. However, we know now that what actually happens is that the hamstring muscles (the muscles in the back of the leg) go into spasm, thus curtailing forward motion (extension). We don't know exactly why this happens, but it is believed to be some kind of protective mechanism.

Laboratory Tests

X ray.   An X ray will only show whether a joint space has narrowed due to the almost complete destruction of articular cartilage; it will not show meniscal damage per se. However, it may reveal calcification of the cartilage—a disorder called *chondrocalcinosis*—which is usually indicative of a degenerative meniscus, which may be prone to tears.

MRI.   An MRI is the test that is most often used to diagnose meniscal injuries. It has a 90 percent accuracy rate for the meniscus, which means it is good but not perfect. On an MRI the meniscus should appear absolutely black. A tear or injury to the meniscus shows up as tiny dots. A tear that is incomplete is classified as a grade 1 or 2. A complete tear through the top and bottom, such as the parrot beak or bucket handle, is classified as grade 3. An MRI should be interpreted by an experienced knee surgeon or orthopedic radiologist; a general radiologist may not be able to distinguish between a grade 2 or 3 tear with the same degree of accuracy as someone who performs a lot of knee surgeries. Generally speaking, a grade 1 or even a grade 2 tear is not considered serious, nor is it apparent through an arthroscopic examination. This tear is probably insignificant as far as causing any symptoms. If the patient is no longer in pain, the physician may conclude that the meniscus has a stable tear that may not be causing any symptoms. Therefore, the physician may decide to forego surgery in favor of a good muscle-strengthening program. If at a later date, the tear worsens and the patient experiences pain, surgery may be reconsidered.

Under the best of circumstances, the MRI is not infallible, and about 10 percent of the time, an MRI will show a grade 2 tear that is actually a more serious grade 3 and vice versa. Therefore, it is very important for the physician to consider carefully the patient's symptoms before making the diagnosis. If the physician is convinced that the patient has a serious tear that will require surgical repair or resection, she will probably decide to arthroscope the knee.

Arthroscopy. An arthroscope by an experienced arthroscopist can achieve an accuracy rate of about 100 percent. From the arthroscope, the physician can determine if a tear is significant and whether it needs surgical repair.

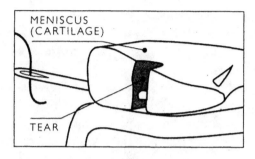

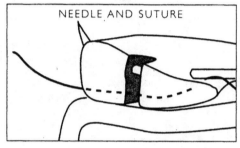

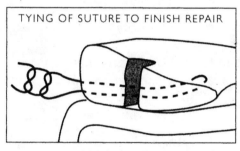

MENISCAL REPAIR

Treating Meniscal Problems

Surgery

The goal of meniscal surgery is to relieve the patient's pain and discomfort and to save as much of the meniscus as possible. The choice of surgery depends on the age of the patient and the location of the meniscal injury. The following procedures can be performed arthroscopically.

Suturing　　　If the patient is young and if the injury is in an area of the meniscus with good blood supply, it is reasonable to resuture the meniscus. This can be performed arthroscopically and, thanks to the most recent technologies, can often be done without a secondary incision. Sutures are passed through a special disposable needle, and then using a knot tying instrument, the knot is passed right onto the cartilage. Multiple sutures are inserted. If the knee has a stable anterior and posterior cruciate ligament, there is an approximate 80 percent chance of healing. The anesthesia can be either local, regional, or general.

Resecting　　　If the patient is elderly or the tear is in an area that does have a good blood supply, the physician may cut off as small a portion of the meniscus as possible to even out the surfaces.

After Surgery

After either surgery, most patients experience pain for a very short interval, and most will be able to return to a desk-type job within 24 hours. Rehabilitation, whether done individually or with a therapist, should begin the day after surgery.

Experimental Therapies

Experiments involving replacing torn or injured menisci with artificial ones have been abysmal failures, and there is virtually no encouraging research being done in this area at the present time. One of the more interesting areas of research involves replacing a previously removed meniscus with a meniscus from a cadaver (allograft). However, the procedure is still highly experimental and, unfortunately, hasn't been very successful. The problem is, the transplanted meniscus can shrink and also tear easily. In fact, in one study involving dogs, the meniscus was surgically removed from each dog and resutured back to the same dog. The results were not good: 70 percent of the dogs were unable to accept back their own meniscus after it had been removed. Much more research is needed in this area before allografts become a viable option.

Rehabilitation Training for Meniscal Repairs

In the past, rehabilitation after meniscal repairs severely limited weight-bearing activities, forcing the patient to use crutches for about 6 weeks after surgery. We have since learned that restricting these activities can actually hamper a patient's recovery. Thus, immediately following surgery, we now allow patients to walk without crutches, bend their legs, and begin leg-strengthening exercises, such as weight lifting, to build up the quadriceps and hamstring muscle groups. When patients regain strength equal in both legs, which usually takes about 6 to 12 weeks, they can return to sports.

The goal of meniscal rehabilitation is to strengthen the muscles of the lower limbs without putting excess strain on the injured meniscus. Stretching the leg muscles (quadriceps, hamstrings, and gastrocnemius) is important because it will promote flexibility (the ease of movement), which is the foundation for maximum strengthening. For specific exercises for meniscal rehabilitation, see page 171.

Injuries to the Articular Cartilage

The articular cartilage is a special type of connective tissue that lines the three bones that form the knee joint—the patella, the femur, and the tibia—and allows the joint to move in a fluid motion. Without this protective layer of articular cartilage, the bones forming the joint would rub together, which could cause a great deal of pain and discomfort, as occurs in arthritis. Also known as *hyaline cartilage,* articular cartilage consists of a white elastic material, similar to the gristle found inside the joint of a turkey leg, and is anywhere from 1/8 to 1/2 inch in thickness.

Articular cartilage consists primarily of water, collagen,

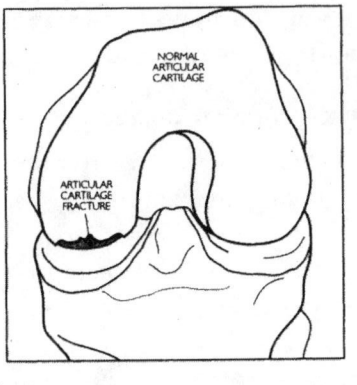
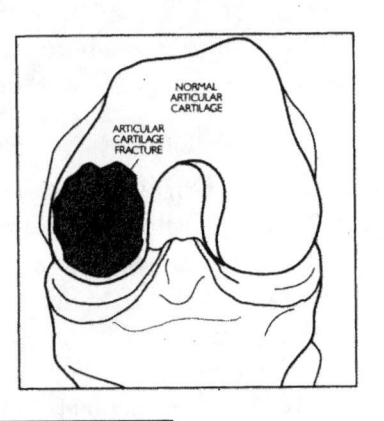
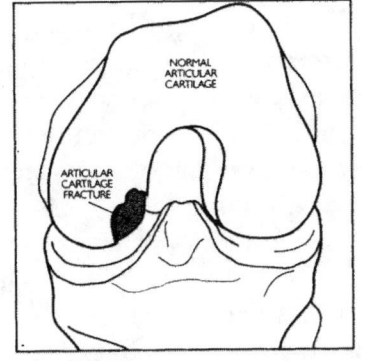

OSTEOCHONDRAL FRACTURES

and other molecules known as *proteoglycans*. Articular cartilage is extremely resilient and is designed so that it can withstand both shear (side) and compression force. This special
cartilage can sustain the enormous force exerted through the
knee when you are running on pavement (which could be up
to seven times your body weight!) or when you are twisting or
pivoting in a sideways motion.

Articular cartilage may be a biomechanical wonder, but it is
not immune to injury from overuse or abuse. In fact, injuries
to the articular cartilage are the most common knee injury.
There is some evidence that continual stress on the articular
cartilage may make it more prone to injury. In addition, over

time, the articular cartilage can simply wear out. In fact, by middle age, nearly everyone will show some degree of damage to their articular cartilage, and if this damage becomes severe enough, it may develop into arthritis. In fact, all forms of arthritis—from the inflammatory variety such as rheumatoid arthritis to "wear-and-tear" osteoarthritis—involve destruction of the articular cartilage.

Problems involving the articular cartilage are one of the most frustrating in all of medicine. Unlike ligament or meniscal injuries, once the articular cartilage is damaged, there is little that can be done. Unfortunately, articular cartilage cannot be replaced or made synthetically. Although not from lack of trying, researchers have been stymied in their attempts to stimulate the body to make it on its own. There are some treatments, however, that I will discuss later in this chapter that may make patients more comfortable and some promising new ones that may actually help the body to better heal itself.

There are four basic types of injuries involving articular cartilage.

Chondral fracture. If you fall directly on your knee or bang your knee very hard, it could result in a fracture of the

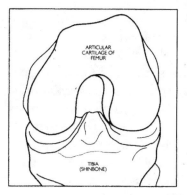

BENT LEFT KNEE FROM FRONT

articular cartilage that does not involve bone. The knee may feel painful and swollen. In this case, the articular cartilage may not be permanently damaged, rather it may simply have become compressed—similar to the way plastic can bend under pressure—and will return to its normal shape immediately. However, there might still be microscopic parts of the articular cartilage that are permanently damaged. The pain is variable and often does not reflect the extent of the injury. Because articular cartilage has no nerve endings, the pain is secondary to abnormal stress placed on the bone that the articular cartilage covers—the subchondral bone. The normal forces of daily activity become abnormal because the shock absorber is damaged. The bone is subsequently stressed, and the patient might experience pain. Fortunately, the bone will eventually remodel itself to withstand the new stress, and the pain will subside, but it could take up to 6 months in some patients.

An MRI cannot "see" articular cartilage, but it will show a tremendous amount of hyperemia, or blood flow, to the injured area, which suggests a chondral fracture.

Chondromalacia.   *Chondromalacia* refers to the softening of the articular cartilage. Articular cartilage is arbitrarily graded from 0 to 4, 0 being normal and 4 being the most damaged. A healthy, smooth surface—the kind that would be found in an uninjured surface—is graded 0. Grade 1 means that there is some blistering or disturbance on the surface; grade 2, the surface is scratched or fissured; grade 3, the fissuring is deeper, almost down to bone; grade 4, the surface is worn away to the bone and the bone is also worn out.

Arbitrarily, if there is destruction to the articular cartilage surface and its appearance to the naked eye is indistinguishable, the terminology is different depending on the patient's age. In those patients under thirty, damage is termed *chondromalacia grade 0 to 4*, whereas over thirty years of age, it is called *osteoarthritis*.

We still have a lot to learn about articular cartilage, but it appears that once the surface is damaged, it is more vulnerable to repetitive wear and tear, destruction, and overuse phenomena. Professional hockey and basketball players invariably have abrasive wearing of the articular cartilage due to the magnitude of the forces and the repetitive nature of the activities involved in their careers. Amateur athletes similarly might suffer from overuse wear and tear, which is technically arthritis.

Traumatic chondromalacia. A significant blow to the knee, such as one that might occur in a football injury, could tear off either a small piece of articular cartilage or a large fragment containing a piece of bone directly under the subchondral surface. This is called an osteochondral fracture. Such a severe injury would cause much discomfort, and if the bone fragment is visible on X ray, it might require surgery.

Osteoarthritis. In older patients, pain and perhaps swelling of the knee in the absence of other injuries could suggest osteoarthritis, a condition that is caused by the gradual wearing down of the articular cartilage.

Diagnosis

If you have swelling and/or pain in your knee, your doctor will look for several causes, including destruction of the articular cartilage. Unfortunately, there is no noninvasive diagnostic test that provides a good view of articular cartilage; only an arthroscope of the area can provide a definitive answer. Very often, we try to rule out other possible problems that we can diagnose using noninvasive methods before considering the articular cartilage.

An X Ray

An X ray will not show the articular cartilage per se, but a standing X ray will show if the spaces between the joints have narrowed, which suggests an erosion of articular cartilage.

MRI

Although I believe that MRI will eventually be able to "see" articular cartilage, to date, it does not with any degree of accuracy. However, it does show whether the menisci are injured or whether any of the ligaments are torn. In addition, an MRI will show whether any bones are bruised, which could indirectly be a sign of injury to the articular cartilage.

Arthroscopy

Your physician may decide to arthroscope the knee to assess the extent of the damage or if he is convinced that there is a problem with the articular cartilage (or any other structure of the knee) that may be improved through surgical intervention.

Treatment

Nonsteroidal Anti-inflammatory Drugs (NSAIDs)

If you are in a great deal of pain and discomfort, your physician may recommend use of NSAIDs. (See Chapter 4 on controlling pain.) I personally believe that medication is a short-term solution, and other steps must be taken to correct this problem.

Exercise

When a joint is injured, the knee begins to swell, which can hamper the movement of the knee and can cause the muscles to atrophy or weaken, placing more force on the joint at a time when it is least able to sustain it. Therefore, it is very important to get the joint moving as soon as possible and to keep the muscles strong. For articular cartilage problems such as arthritis or chondromalacia, I recommend a low-impact exercise program that strengthens the muscles without stressing the joint (see page 171 for details). Activities such as swimming, riding a stationary bicycle, or even using a cross-country ski machine could be beneficial. (If you use a stationary bicycle, set the seat in such a way so that you do not bend you knee more than 90 degrees, because it often causes discomfort.) If you are disciplined about exercising, you may work out on your own. However, if you exercise haphazardly, you may need to work out with a trainer or at an exercise rehabilitation center. In this world of medical cost containment, there will unquestionably be a cutback in rehabilitative services, so that patients will be required to exercise on their own.

"Washing Out" the Joint

Very often, a patient with an injured joint may have difficulty extending her leg and keeps the knee in a flexed position. This is often due to a protective spasm of the hamstrings, and gentle exercise may help return the leg to normal motion. However, a "locked" leg may also result from a torn or jagged piece of cartilage that is caught in the joint (either between the tibia and the femur or the patella and the femur) and is preventing full extension. If your doctor suspects that this is the case, he may arthroscope the knee to "wash out" the debris and smooth out the surface. Although this isn't a permanent solution, many patients feel better.

Reattaching the Cartilage

If a big piece of articular cartilage with its underlying bone is ripped off in an injury, it may be possible to reattach it back into position using wires or absorbable pins. If indeed, there is a significant bone attached, the injury is an osteochondral fracture, and if there is a short interval (roughly 4 to 8 weeks) between injury and surgery, there is an excellent chance that the fracture will heal if pinned back into position. If the injury does not include a bone surface, the articular cartilage by itself cannot be reattached with any certainty of success. Instead, attention is directed to the bone to produce fibrocartilage, which, although biomechanically inferior to articular cartilage, will fill the defect.

It would be wonderful if there was a synthetic material that could be used to "paint" back missing areas of articular cartilage. Unfortunately, there is nothing comparable that is available now. Although investigation and experimentation is being done, today there are only three methods of replacing absent cartilage:

- Procedures designed to stimulate or regenerate the growth of cartilage cells.
- Bulk allografts (bone transplants).
- Cartilage cell growth and subsequent transplantation.

Regeneration of Cartilage.   Since the 1800s, scientists have dreamed of developing a way to get the body to regenerate articular cartilage, and although there have been some promising developments in this field, it is still highly experimental. In the body, cartilage is produced by special cells that, depending on their location, have the ability to produce either bone, fibrous tissue, or cartilage. We don't know the precise triggers that "turn on" these cells and instruct them to produce cartilage. We do know, however, that injuring the bone can in many cases trigger the growth of cartilage. There are several ways that we do this, but basically they all involve making the bone bleed. In some cases, the surgeon will drill holes in the bone to stimulate these special cells to grow cartilage. Another procedure called *abrasion arthroplasty* involves a more aggressive procedure that causes more bleeding and hopefully produces more fibrocartilage. All of these procedures to stimulate fibrocartilage production can be done arthroscopically, but because the bone is actually involved, the procedures are associated with more discomfort than routine arthroscopy.

Bulk Allografts. Bulk allografts are pieces of bone and/or cartilage that are taken from a cadaver and put in the patient. For years, this procedure has been done in tumor patients. Unfortunately, many of these cancer patients also underwent chemotherapy and radiation treatments and thus were immunosuppressed, which made them prone to infection. As a result, there was a rather significant complication rate—as high as 50 percent—including severe infection, possibly requiring amputation.

The use of bulk allografts for cartilage transplantation in nonimmunosuppressed patients should result in a lower complication rate. As of this writing, however, there are too few cases to collect any significant data.

Cell Transplantation. Cell transplantation is another experimental method of replacing lost articular cartilage that has received a great deal of publicity lately. In this procedure, cartilage cells are taken from the patient and then cultured in the laboratory. The cells multiply, producing an abundance of cartilage, and then are reintroduced surgically into the patient. Theoretically, cell transplantation will heal, thus restoring the surface with normal articular cartilage. This experimental procedure was recently reported in the Scandanavian medical literature. The results were promising; however, the patient population was small and primarily had minor defects on either the patellar–femoral or tibia surface. The femoral surface defects appeared to do better than the tibial defects. As exciting as this new procedure may be, it leads many unanswered questions including: How big a defect can be filled? Will it be applicable to all three compartments—the patellar–femoral, the medial femoral–tibial, and the lateral femoral–tibial? Will the patient be able to return to sports? Only time and experience will answer these questions.

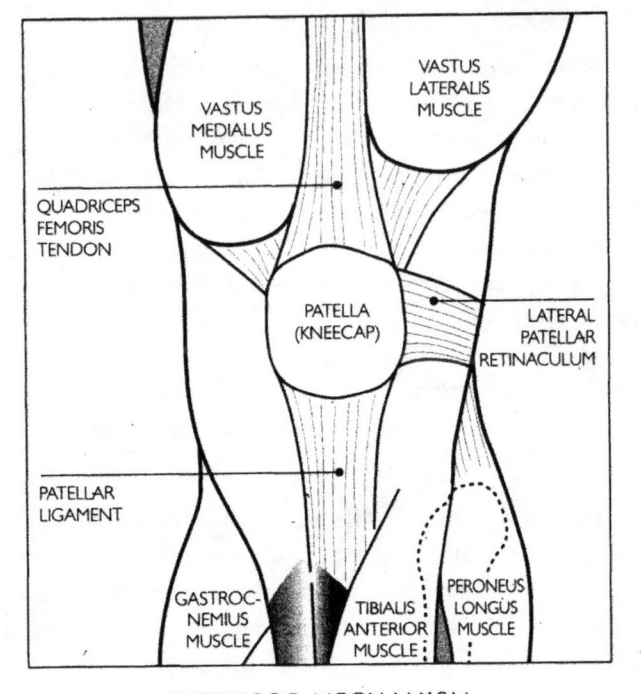

EXTENSOR MECHANISM

Patella Injuries

The patella—also called the kneecap—is a small, flat triangular bone that is located on the front of the knee. It is only 2 to 3 inches wide, yet it is a critical part of the extensor mechanism, the group of muscles, tendons, and ligaments that work together to make it possible to straighten the leg and perform such essential activities as standing and walking. Because the patella is such an integral part of the extensor mechanism, we often use the broader label of extensor mechanism discomfort to describe patella-related problems.

The extensor mechanism consists of the quadriceps muscles, the quadriceps tendon, the patella, the patellar tendon, the tibial tubercle, and the lateral and medial retiniculum.

From the top of the knee, the quadriceps muscles hold the patella against the femur, or thigh bone. From the side, the patella is held in place by fibrous bands called *retinicula*. From the bottom of the knee, the patella is connected to the tibia via the patellar tendon. The back of the patella is covered with the thickest layer of articular cartilage of any joint in the body, which gives the patella special properties.

The patella moves as the leg moves—it glides up and down, and rotates on the femur until it's in its track, the trochlea. The patella helps to keep the knee joint properly aligned, and it is also important for muscle strength by giving the quadriceps the extra leverage they need to cope with the enormous force that runs through the knee with each step or run. In fact, if the patella is removed, the force of extension is reduced by about 30 percent, which severely hampers the efficiency of the quadriceps and increases the force exerted through the joint. The patella also cushions and protects the other bones of the joint. For example, in the case of a fall or blow to the knee, the patella may prevent the condyles (bony knobs) of the tibia or femur from being injured.

Nonspecific knee pain or extensor mechanism pain is one of the most common complaints among patients. (Your doctor may refer to it as anterior knee pain or extensor mechanism discomfort.) It is characterized by a dull ache while walking up stairs or squatting, or the knee may suddenly give way or may catch when flexing. Very often, patients complain of grating and creaking when they extend or flex their knee or discomfort after sitting in one spot for a long time, such as when watching a movie.

At one time, kneecap pain was routinely diagnosed as chondromalacia, which is really a pathological condition characterized by the softening and progressive breakdown of articular cartilage. However, autopsy studies and surgery of patients without knee pain have shown that chondromalacia is very common, particularly among older people and, in most cases, does not cause problems. Therefore, we now use the

broader term of *anterior knee pain* to describe patellar discomfort. What precisely does cause patellar pain? There are
several potential culprits.

Chondromalacia

Chondromalacia, one of the most common causes of knee
pain in younger people, can be caused by a traumatic injury to
the patella, such as a severe blow, but can sometimes occur for
no apparent reason. Chondromalacia also appears to be part
of the normal aging process. In fact, in older people, the
wearing away of articular cartilage is called *osteoarthritis*.
However—and this is what's confusing for so many patients—
there is no evidence that chondromalacia in younger people
will lead to arthritis down the road. We used to assume that
chondromalacia in the young would automatically develop
into arthritis. However, careful studies have shown that there
is no clear-cut progression. In fact, we now believe that although the end result is the same, chondromalacia and arthritis may be very different problems caused by different
circumstances. In addition, there is no direct correlation between patellar pain and destruction caused by chondromalacia. Sometimes a person with mild symptoms can actually
have more destruction than someone who is in constant pain.

Chondromalacia is rated according to the severity of the
condition on a scale of 0 to grade 4, with 0 considered healthy,
smooth cartilage. In grade 1 chondromalacia, there is some
blistering or disturbance on the surface of the articular cartilage; grade 2 chondromalacia, the surface is scratched or fissured; grade 3 chondromalacia, the fissuring is deeper or
down to the bone; grade 4 chondromalacia, the surface is
worn away down to the bone and the bone is also worn out.

The pain caused by chondromalacia is somewhat mysteri-
ous, because there are no nerve endings in the articular cartilage. However, it is believed that when the articular cartilage is

damaged to the point that it is no longer an efficient shock absorber, the force exerted through the bones, which are rich in nerve endings, is all the greater. We perceive the extra force as pain.

Chondromalacia is usually diagnosed by symptoms. An X ray will not show chondromalacia. An arthroscope will conclusively show the presence of chondromalacia and the stage of the disease. However, if your doctor suspects that chondromalacia is the problem, he will probably prescribe a good strengthening program since there is little that can be done surgically to improve the situation. In some cases, the surgeon may wash out the area, that is, smooth the surface of the articular cartilage (on the back of the patella) and remove any debris that may be causing the joint to "catch." Patients are also usually advised to refrain from activities that may aggravate the pain. (For more information on treatment of problems related to the articular cartilage, see page 100.)

Abnormal Kneecap Alignment

Ideally, the kneecap should lie directly under the quadriceps in the center of the knee. In some people, however, the kneecap sits slightly off to one side or the other. In women, for example, the kneecap sits off to the side toward the center of the body, making women somewhat knock-kneed. To accommodate a woman's wider pelvis, the femur is angled toward the other leg and the tibia is angled outward. On the other hand, many men are bowlegged, in which the femur angles inward as does the tibia. In fact, between 30 and 40 percent of the population—primarily women—has some kind of an abnormal knee alignment. In some cases, a malalignment of the kneecap can pull it off track. However, a trauma such as a twisting injury can also knock the kneecap off its track. If the kneecap partially comes off its track, its called a *subluxation.* If the kneecap is entirely off track—for example, it sits way off

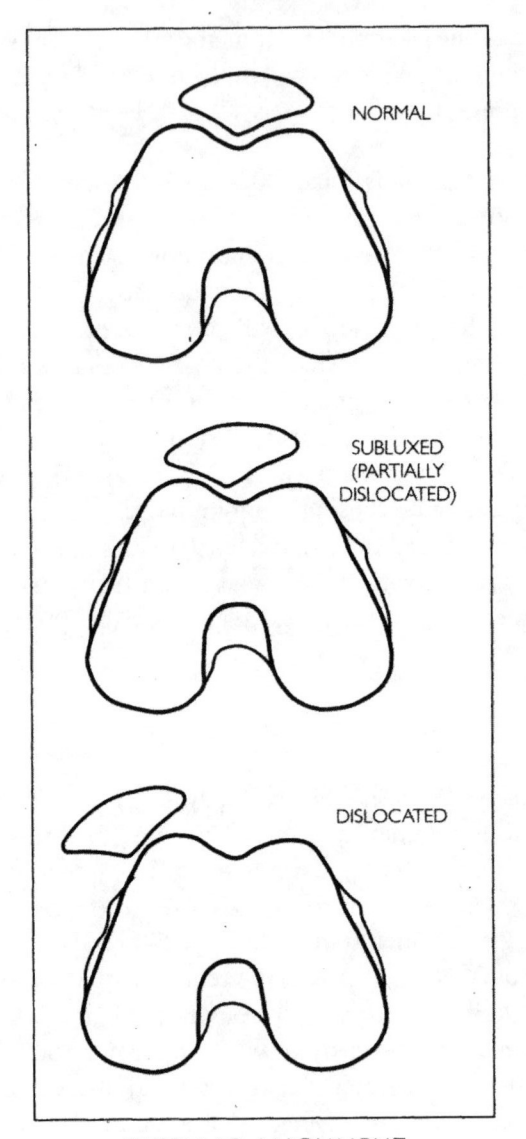

NORMAL

SUBLUXED
(PARTIALLY
DISLOCATED)

DISLOCATED

PATELLAR ALIGNMENT

to the side instead of in the center—it's called a *dislocation.* Although some people may not be bothered at all by irregular alignment, others may experience discomfort. Very often, the problem can often be corrected by strengthening the surrounding leg muscles, thus improving their shock-absorbing ability. I advise patients to try a well-supervised rehabilitation program for 6 months before seeking further treatment. However, if the patient is in a great deal of pain and a good rehabilitation program has not helped, surgical correction may be considered.

Treatment

Surgery

Kneecap alignment problems can be diagnosed by X ray, which will clearly show a patella that is off track. Depending on the cause of the problem, the following types of surgery may be performed.

Lateral Release.   In some cases, the patella is being pulled off track by tight lateral bands, or retinaculum, which the physician can feel when she palpates the area. In a lateral release, which is done arthroscopically, the surgeon simply cuts the lateral bands, reducing the lateral pull on the patella, thus the patella moves back into place.

As with any arthroscopic procedure, possible risks include a small chance of developing an infection (under 1 percent), nerve damage, skin numbness, and other problems that are described on your patient consent form, which all patients should read carefully.

Patellar Realignment.   There are two types of surgical procedures for patellar realignment: proximal realignment or distal realignment.

In a proximal realignment, an open-knee procedure, the surgeon must first perform a lateral release. After the lateral release, he cuts a piece of the quadriceps tendon (all the way down around the medial side of the patella to the medial border of the patellar tendon) and resutures the quadriceps tendon to a more medial position.

In a distal realignment (which may also include a proximal realignment), the surgeon moves the patellar tendon insertion at the tibia tubercle over to a more medial position and sometimes distal and elevated.

Exercise

Rehabilitation is crucial after patellar surgery. Keep in mind that surgery is not a cure-all. Even after surgery, it is imperative that you continue with a good strengthening program tailored your particular problem.

Bracing

Some people may find that a functional brace worn during activity may offer some relief for patellar problems. Frankly, there is no specific evidence that it does; however, it may have a subtle effect on the tracking of the kneecap, which could relieve discomfort. A patellar femoral workout brace is primarily a sleeve made of cloth or neoprene (rubber). This brace has a hole or pad around the kneecap to stress-relieve the area. A different variety of the patella brace has single straps around the distal (lower) part of the extensor mechanism around the patellar tendon. Either brace is fine if it works for you. Avoid braces that are too tight around the kneecap or an Ace bandage that compresses the knee too tightly—both can cause further discomfort. Braces can be purchased at surgical supply stores and some sporting good stores.

Other Possibilities

Patellar Fractures

A hard blow to the patella could result in a bone fracture, and due to the small size of the patella, it can be very difficult to repair. The standard methods of bone repair, open reduction and internal fixation—using wires and screws to put a bone back in place—is not easily performed on a bone that is roughly 2 to 3 inches in diameter. There is always a risk that if the surgical repair doesn't work, it could actually cause more problems. The problems are secondary to the postoperative problems that are attendant to the immobilization required for fracture healing. The patient might have to be casted for upward of 6 weeks, which could result in stiffness. However, since the patella is such a critical part of the extensor mechanism, we try very hard to save it when we can. This is really dependent on whether the fracture is comminuted (in multiple pieces) or has one or two large pieces. In some cases we can't save the patella, and it must be removed. After patella surgery, it is essential to get the joint moving again as soon as possible, because if it is immobile even for a short period, the joint will become stiff.

Osteochondritis Dessicans of the Patella or the Trochlea

Osteochondritis dessicans is a rare condition that primarily strikes children. For some unknown reason, the blood supply to a particular portion of bone is cut off, resulting in the death of the particular bone. The bone either falls off, which requires surgical reattachment or removal, or it may reattach itself and heal on its own. In the case of osteochondritis dessicans of the patella or trochlea, the articular cartilage on the surface of the patella or the trochlea can be disrupted, resulting in pain. Osteochondritis dessicans is diagnosed by X ray and the symptoms are pain and sometimes locking is possible if the piece of bone falls off.

Patellar–femoral Arthritis

Isolated patellar–femoral arthritis is a very rare condition. More often than not, arthritis will affect the entire joint, that is, the three compartments: the patellar–femoral, the medial femoral–tibial, and the lateral femoral–tibial. It will not stay confined to one compartment. In fact, according to one cadaver study, only 4 percent had isolated patellar–femoral arthritis, and women with kneecap malalignment were more prone to this problem. Patellar–femoral arthritis is difficult to treat. In cases of more generalized arthritis, if the disease becomes so severe that there is significant raw bone causing a great deal of pain, the physician may recommend a total knee replacement, which involves the resurfacing of all the bones of the knee joint with a prosthesis. However, if only the patella is arthritic, there are few options. Surgery involving only a patellar–femoral replacement—that is, the surgeon resurfaces only the patella and the trochlea of the femur—has not been that successful. In fact, there is less than a 50 percent chance that it will work as compared to a 95 percent success rate for a total knee replacement. However, because the arthritis has not affected other sites, physicians are reluctant to perform a total knee replacement, which in that situation would require the removal of healthy bone and articular cartilage. Usually, in the case of patellar–femoral arthritis, physicians will encourage their patients to undertake a serious strengthening program to see if that can relieve some of the pain. If the patient is over fifty-five, the exercise program is not working, and the patient is absolutely miserable, the physician may recommend a total knee replacement.

Rehabilitation Training for Patellar–Femoral-Type Syndrome

Similar to rehabilitation training for arthritis, the basic exercise plan for kneecap pain is to minimize weight-bearing stress while strengthening the surrounding muscles to assist normal patella tracking. For specific exercises for patellar rehabilitation, see page 171.

Ligament Injuries

It was the funniest sensation. What happened was, one minute I was skiing down a mountain and went to turn to the right but the edge of my ski got stuck. I felt a pop, fell to the ground, and then began to have pain. I didn't have a clue as to what happened. I tried to get up and walk, but my knee just sort of dissolved.

Ann, forty-seven, accountant,
suffered injury of the anterior cruciate
and medial collateral ligaments

Ligaments are strong, fibrous bands of tissue that connect bones to bones. The main function of ligaments is to stabilize the joint while at the same time allowing for movement. Without the ligaments holding the bones in place, your knees would be weak and wobbly. The simplest movement—getting up from a chair or even walking across the room—would be impossible.

The knee bones are connected to each other by several groups of ligaments. There are basically four major ligaments of the knee that keep the bones in check: the medial collateral ligament (MCL), the lateral collateral ligament (LCL), the anterior cruciate ligament (ACL), and the posterior cruciate ligament (PCL). The other ligaments are really part of the thick capsule that encases the knee. These other ligaments—the deep MCL, the posterior oblique ligament, the oblique popliteal ligament—are not primary but secondary stabilizers.

The cruciate ligaments are intraarticular ligaments, which means they are deep inside the joint and cannot be felt from the outside. The collateral ligaments are extraarticular ligaments, which means they are situated on the outside of the joint and can be felt through the skin. Each of these ligaments has its own specific function, although there is some overlap, and each is vulnerable to injury under the right conditions.

A ligament that is injured in a chronic situation can be stretched beyond its normal elasticity like a worn-out rubber band, or it can actually be torn apart in an acute injury. When a ligament is stretched or torn, it is called a *sprain*. A knee sprain may occur if you suddenly pivot or twist too far in one direction, thus pulling on the ligament, or a sprain can also occur from a sudden twist or blow to the knee. A knee sprain can be very minor—you may feel nothing more than slight discomfort—or it can be serious and painful, depending on the ligament involved and the extent of the injury.

The Collateral Ligaments

The MCL is a broad, thick band located on the inside of the knee; it runs down the inside of the knee from the femur to the tibia and has two parts. One part is the deep MCL, which is really a condensation of the thick capsule and is the most substantial and biggest component of the MCL, and the second part is the superficial MCL, which extends about 4 to 6 inches down the inside of the tibia. Its primary function is to prevent the leg from hinging open, but it is also part of the mechanism that allows the knee to rotate. The MCL is vulnerable to blows from the lateral side (typical of contact sports such as football), which can overstretch the ligament on the inside of the knee, resulting in injury.

Thinner than the MCL, the LCL runs down the outside of the leg and is not particularly vulnerable to injury, unless by chance you are struck by a blow on the inside of your knee, resulting in a stretching of the LCL. The LCL connects the femur to the fibula, the small bone that runs down the side of the knee. Similar to the MCL, the LCL has a stabilizing function in that it prevents the knee from collapsing in and also is involved in rotation of the knee.

Diagnosis Tests

Physical Examination.   The physician will check for pain or tenderness along the course of the ligament.

Tests for Stability.   To determine whether one of the collateral ligaments is sprained, your physician will exert pressure on the outside or the inside of the straight and or slightly bent knee, reproducing the mechanism of injury. Depending on the degree of pain or the looseness of the joint, the sprain will be classified as follows: A grade 1 sprain, the least serious injury, involves some tenderness and discomfort at the point of the injury. A grade 2 sprain also involves pain and tenderness, but the knee actually will open up on examination to about 5 millimeters. In a grade 3 sprain, the knee will open up as far as 1 centimeter, which can produce substantial instability. A grade 3 sprain is almost invariably associated with a torn ACL.

MRI.   MRI has a greater than 90 percent accuracy in diagnosing injuries to the collateral ligaments and in assessing the seriousness of these sprains. X rays will not be helpful unless the ligament sprain is associated with an avulsion of a piece of bone.

Treatment

Grade 1, 2, and 3 sprains will all heal without surgery. Because there is very little, if any, instability with either a grade 1 or 2, healing is very predictable. Grade 3 tears, however, are often associated with ACL tears and might not heal if there is an instability that develops because the ACL and collateral ligaments are injured.

Exercise.   At one time, it was common practice to immobilize the leg by casting it for up to 6 weeks, but we now try to encourage movement as early as possible. The leg may be immobilized for a brief period of time (usually 72 hours) simply to relieve the pain. Ice and analgesics may be used to reduce pain and swelling. After a few days, the patient is started on rehabilitative therapy to get the knee moving. For the patient's comfort, the physician may also prescribe a small sleeve-type brace to be worn on the knee, but it is not necessary for stability. Recovery for a grade 1 sprain may take up to 10 days, and a grade 2 sprain could take up to 4 weeks.

A grade 3 sprain is treated differently in that there is some controversy in the orthopedic community as to whether a grade 3 sprain can actually exist without concurrent damage to one of the cruciate ligaments, usually the ACL. If the ACL is involved, the usual treatment involves surgical reconstruction of the ACL (which is discussed later in this chapter) along with a prescribed program of exercise therapy. In the rare case in which an MRI will clearly show a perfect ACL along with a grade 3 sprain of a collateral ligament, the physician may treat the problem the same way he would a grade 1 or 2 sprain.

Prevention

Exercise.   The best way to prevent injuries to either one of the collateral ligaments is to develop muscle strength in your legs. The stronger the quadriceps and hamstring muscles, the less likely you are to sustain a severe injury of the collateral ligaments.

Bracing.   In recent years, there has been some debate over the value of wearing a protective brace while engaging in contact sports such as football. Many coaches swear by braces and claim that they can prevent ligament injuries. There are little scientific data to support this belief, and more studies are underway to determine if wearing a brace can prevent injuries or can prevent a recurrence after a previous injury. Until we have the facts, I don't believe that we can make a definitive judgment on bracing; however, based on current studies, it doesn't appear to hurt to wear one. Just keep in mind that a brace is not magic armor, and you still need to exercise caution.

Cruciate Ligaments

The cruciate ligaments—so named because they crisscross each other—are embedded deep inside the knee joint. The ACL, which connects the femur to the tibia, is only 2 inches in length and ¾ inch in width, but it is critical in helping to maintain stability. The ACL limits rotation of the knee and restricts the forward motion of the tibia. There are between 100,000 and 250,000 ACL injuries each year. It is more prone to injury than other ligaments and can be stretched or torn by a sudden twisting or torquing motion. For example, losing control of your skis or landing improperly during a basketball game (in which your feet go one way and your knee is turned another way) can result in an injured ACL.

A torn ACL may or may not hurt at the time of injury, depending on the type of injury. Very often, a patient will talk about hearing a pop and suddenly finding that her leg has literally buckled under. Depending on the extent of the injury, stiffness and swelling may persist for some time. In the case of a minor stretch or tear, the injury may resolve itself; however, if the tear is significant, an injured ACL can severely curtail activity.

The PCL is about 2 inches long and slightly wider than the ACL. It connects the femur to the tibia. This ligament restricts the backward motion of the leg and is rarely injured in sports but may be ripped or torn as a result of a traumatic injury such as an automobile accident.

Diagnosis

Physical Examination. Palpating, or feeling, the knee in conjunction with stability testing are the primary ways that a physician can make a quick assessment of an injury without surgical intervention. However, because the cruciate ligaments are deep inside the knee, the physician can't palpate the area for pain or tenderness. Therefore, unlike tears of the collateral ligaments, which can be graded according to severity (grade 1, the least serious, to grade 3, the most serious), cruciate ligaments cannot be graded in a similar fashion because they cannot be felt.

Stability Tests.   The Lachman test (see page 29) is often used to test the ACL. In this test, the doctor puts the leg in full extension and then pulls the tibia forward, almost as if he's trying to pull the tibia away. If the leg moves 5 millimeters or more from the right to left, it could signify a torn ACL. A KT test quantifies the displacement with a Lachman test. The KT is a handheld machine placed on the tibia as the physician performs the test.

An anterior drawer test is also used to assess the integrity of the ACL. The knee is bent 90 degrees, and the physician pulls the tibia forward. If it moves more than 5 millimeters forward, it strongly suggests a torn ACL.

The posterior drawer test is used to test the PCL. In this test, the physician bends the knee 90 degrees and pushes the tibia back. If the leg moves more than 5 millimeters backward, it strongly suggests a torn PCL.

MRI.   An MRI has an accuracy of almost 90 percent in determining a normal or completely torn ACL or PCL. Normally, the ACL or PCL appears as a dark structure that runs from the corresponding origin to its insertion. The MRI, however, is not very good in detailing a partial tear. The partial tear can be diagnosed by arthroscopy.

Arthroscopy.   During arthroscopy, the physician can gently pull the ACL to determine the degree of injury and whether it warrants further treatment. However, this is very subjective, and much of the diagnosis depends on the skill and experience of the surgeon.

Treatment

The ACL.   There are two courses of treatment for ACL injuries, the nonoperative approach and surgery.

- *Nonoperative*   The physician and patient may opt to try an exercise strengthening program in lieu of surgery.
- *Surgery*   The ACL is surgically reconstructed, and the patient is then put into a rehabilitation program.

The treatment approach depends primarily on the injury and the lifestyle and goals of the patient and any other associated injuries, for example, a concurrent torn collateral ligament or meniscal tear.

Only one-third of all people with a completely torn ACL will be able to build up their muscle strength to the point that they will be able to resume normal activity without surgery. In time, these lucky few will be able to run, jump, ski, play basketball—in short, do whatever they want—with little more than a functional knee brace for added support. The odds of success through exercise alone are not as good for women as it is for men. Born with less muscle strength than men and looser ligaments, most women will not be able to develop enough muscle strength to compensate for the insufficient ligament.

Sedentary younger people who don't mind curtailing their activities and older, less active people may opt for an exercise strengthening program instead of surgery. Because the injury is not interfering with their lifestyle, there is less urgency to operate. However, an active, athletic person will often choose immediate surgical intervention followed by a rehabilitation program geared at getting her back to full activity as soon as possible.

Lifestyle is only one consideration in choosing treatment; the long-term implications of not surgically correcting the ligament tear is another important factor. Studies show that about 65 percent of all patients with a torn ACL will go on to develop a torn meniscus, which we now know may predispose them to the early onset of arthritis. Although the data are still lacking to directly link a torn ACL with arthritis, the indirect association has been established. Meniscal tears and/or subsequent resection of either all or part of the meniscus in most settings lead to arthritic changes, the primary reason for the trend toward repairing the meniscus. Because 65 percent of people with a torn ACL will eventually develop a torn meniscus, the ACL at least indirectly contributes to the development of arthritis. Consequently, it appears that a reconstruction might play some role in the prevention or minimization of the development of arthritis. The appropriate data, however, necessary to support this hypothesis are still lacking. As the years accumulate, we should eventually have the hard facts to support this assumption.

No matter which treatment option you choose, I want to stress that the recovery process for an ACL injury is not easy. For the patient selecting a nonoperative approach, the rehabilitative process will take approximately 4 months. In fact, the rehabilitative training for a cruciate injury can take anywhere from 3 months to a year and requires a significant time commitment (at least 3 days a week for about 45 minutes each day). However, in most cases, your efforts will be rewarded: surgical intervention along with appropriate rehabilitative training has a success rate of 90 percent, meaning that 90 percent of patients will have a functional knee allowing them to return to their recreational lifestyle.

Surgery

PRIMARY REPAIRS.   It seems logical that if you have a torn ligament, the simplest solution would be to suture or sew it back together, a procedure called a *primary repair*. However, results of resuturing the ligament have been quite dismal. Initially, the patients did well, but over time, the ligament will show symptoms of instability. Reconstruction, or making a new ligament, is now the rule rather than the exception. There is only one situation in which a primary repair of an ACL is appropriate: an avulsion injury in which the ligament remains intact, but it has been pulled off the bone. This type of injury can easily be repaired by simply reattaching the bone avulsion to its previous insertion. An avulsion injury is rare and occurs in skeletally immature individuals (children), whose growth plates are still open. Because the plates are still open—the skeleton is still growing—the attachment to the bone is actually weaker than the ligament itself. Thus the ligament will tear at its weakest link, the attachment to the bone.

RECONSTRUCTION. The most common type of surgery for an ACL injury involves reconstructing the torn ligament with either a healthy tissue (a graft) from the patient, called an *autograft;* a ligament from a cadaver, called an *allograft;* or a synthetic ligament.

An Autograft

The most successful type of reconstructive surgery involves using an autograft, which means that the healthy tissue used to reconstruct the damaged ACL comes from the patient's own body. Typically, the graft is taken from the central one-third of the patellar tendon, which is located just below the kneecap. Although it is less common, the graft can also be taken from the semitendonosis and gracilis tendons, which are located on the inside of the knee. However, studies show that the bone–patellar tendon–bone graft is stronger and heals better and, therefore, whenever possible is the procedure of choice.

Prior to surgery, the patient is given a sedative-hypnotic to induce sleep and then given a general anesthesia. In some cases, depending on the duration of the surgery, the patient might be intubated with a tube and respirator or given a spinal or epidural anesthesia. Patients do not feel anything and are not aware of the surgery.

A small incision (2 to 3 inches) is made to remove the portion of the patellar tendon that is to be grafted. The rest of the procedure is done arthroscopically. The autograft, which becomes the new ACL, is attached to the origin (femur) and inserted to the tibia through drill holes that are cylindrically reproduced to match the size of the bone–tendon–bone graft. The metal screws are a primarily temporary fixation until your own bone fills in and becomes the permanent anchors of the knee. Except in a small percentage of cases, the screws are left in place. In rare cases, one of the screws might become tender to the touch and require removal, which usually would not be done until a year after surgery.

Immediately following the surgery, the new structure is significantly stronger than a normal ACL, but it quickly loses strength as the body begins to fully incorporate the new ligament with the other components of the knee. There are several steps involved in the process of adopting the new ligament to its new location (or, in the case of an allograft, to its new body). First, the body undergoes a process called *revascularization* in which it passes a new blood supply to the ligament. Without an adequate supply of blood, the ligament cannot survive. This critical stage is followed by another important process called the *recollagenization stage*. In recollagenization, the body "changes" the collagen of the reconstructed ligament with that of its own collagen. It takes the body approximately 6 to 12 months to fully accept the new ligament. Unfortunately, during the process, the ligament loses approximately 40 to 50 percent of its initial strength. However, because the transplanted ligament was so much stronger than the normal ACL to begin with, the loss of some strength should not interfere with the patient's ability to return to a functional lifestyle. Although the reconstructed ACL is not a normal ACL, it should be good enough so that the patient can return to a preinjury sports and activity level.

Albeit rare, complications from surgery can include infection (approximately 1 percent); peroneal nerve palsy, which would mean loss of foot function (less than 1 percent); loss of screw fixation at either the tibial or femoral tunnels (less than

1 percent); fracture of the patella (less than 1 percent); and other potential problems that are rare but could make the patient worse.

The gracilis–semitendonosis tendon combination shows a good early result, but with increasing time, this combination does not hold up as well to the bone–patellar tendon–bone combination. This procedure usually requires one incision to harvest the appropriate autograft and several punctures to accommodate the arthroscope and the surgical instruments. It usually lasts less than 2 hours, and most patients are home within 24 hours.

An Allograft

In some cases, a cadaver ligament is used to reconstruct the new ACL, which helps preserve the patient's own patellar tendon. This procedure, which is called an allograft, works almost as well as the *autograft,* but it can take longer to heal microscopically—12 to 18 months as compared to 6 to 12 months. Also, there is some evidence to suggest that the allograft might not be as strong as the autograft and may not yield as good a result.

At one time, grafting cadaver ligaments was risky because screening for human immunodeficiency virus (HIV, the AIDS virus) was not performed. During that era, there was one documented case of HIV transmission due to a cadaver ligament transplant. Today, however, screening techniques and specimen tests for these diseases along with superb sterilization techniques have substantially diminished that risk to what is now approximately 1 in 2 million. Even though the risk is minuscule, to be on the safe side, I believe that allografts should be restricted to patients for whom the benefits clearly outweigh any potential risks. For example, an athletic older patient whose tendon may be weakened by age may fare better with an allograft from a younger person. In addition, if a patient has already used his own patellar tendon and requires a second reconstruction, the best choice might be an allograft.

A Prosthesis

By far, the safest and easiest way to reconstruct an ACL would be simply to use a synthetic or man-made ligament. Unfortunately, synthetic ligaments have such a poor track record that they are rarely used in the United States. In the 1980s, a synthetic ligament made out of Gore-Tex was used in ACL reconstructions. Initially, the synthetic ligament worked well, but the success rate at 5 years was below 50 percent. The man-made ligament could simply not withstand the normal stresses placed on the knee and quickly frayed and broke. A new and supposedly vastly improved version of this ligament is now being used in Canada, and I suspect it will be approved for use in the United States soon. Although the early results are encouraging, it will be several years before we know whether this synthetic ligament can withstand the test of time.

Postsurgery and Recovery

After ACL surgery, you will probably spend between 2 and 3 hours in the recovery room. A large bandage and drain will be put on your elevated knee to control bleeding. The dressing is usually removed the day after surgery. A lightweight brace that allows for motion is worn for up to 2 weeks to protect the knee. You can bear weight on your leg the day of surgery. As soon as possible, you will use a continuous passive motion (CPM) machine, which flexes and extends the leg as you lie in your bed. CPM can help prevent the joint from becoming stiff due to inactivity. You will probably be in pain and will be given pain medication as needed. Ice will also help control pain and swelling. At one time patients used to spend up to 48 hours in the hospital, but most insurance companies are now insisting that patients leave within 24 hours.

Over the next 2 to 3 weeks, you may experience night sweats and a fever of up to 101. This is normal and if you're uncomfortable and your physician agrees, you can bring your fever down with two acetaminophen (Tylenol) or a dose or two of antibiotics to minimize the risk of infection.

In the morning, your knee may feel particularly stiff or painful. An ice pack can help relieve the pain before you begin your therapy.

The average return to sports takes around 6 months, but it can range anywhere between 3 and 12 months, assuming you are diligent about doing your exercises. Your knee will eventually heal with all but a tiny scar remaining. Scar tissue has a tendency to tan darker than normal skin, so if you are out in the sun for a prolonged period of time within the first 12 months after surgery, you might want to cover your knee.

The PCL   PCL injuries are not as well understood as that of the ACL and are currently being studied. As the follow-up studies are becoming available, it becomes apparent that people whose physical examinations or KT evaluations reveal a 1 centimeter or more movement side to side (normal is under 3 millimeters) on a posterior drawer test will probably not do well with an exercise program and will need surgery. The exercise program should stress quadriceps strengthening until both legs are equal in strength. The patients are then healed and can return to their sports. For those whose examination is more than 10 millimeters, a reconstruction using a bone–patellar tendon–bone autograft or allograft or achilles tendon allograft is recommended. To date, there is no consensus of opinion of the superiority of one preparation over the other.

Rehabilitation Training for Ligament Injuries

What I wasn't prepared for was the amount of pain that was involved in getting back flexibility in terms of bending and straightening my knee. It's not easy—you have to make a commitment to therapy. I look at this as

a down payment on being able to do things that I want
to do for the rest of my life.

If I don't do the therapy, if I don't make the effort to
get well, I'm not going to be able to play basketball
with my kids, I'm not going to be able to play tennis
with them. I don't want to be limited—I guess that's
the whole issue.

Joan, thirty-six years old, ACL reconstruction

The typical patient for ACL reconstruction is someone who is very active and whose primary goal is to return to an active lifestyle.

If a patient is not committed to rehabilitation, the surgery will not be successful. The training for ACL recovery can take on average 6 months, at least three days a week for forty-five minutes a session. If possible, anyone contemplating an ACL reconstruction should consult with a physiatrist (a physician who specializes in physical medicine and rehabilitation) or a physical therapist prior to surgery so that he fully understands his role in his recovery. Some insurance companies will cover the cost of rehabilitation; however, given the increasing concerns over cost containment in this country, many patients are forced to do their therapy on their own.

The student or desk worker can return to work within a week following surgery. Patients can resume driving between four and six weeks. Use of pain medicine should be minimal after 3 weeks.

Rehabilitation for an ACL reconstruction should only be done at a center that is experienced in rehabilitating patients with ligament problems and should have special machinery geared for these patients. The staff at advanced centers should have expertise in training techniques to ensure a quick and safe return to maximum function. In addition, a center that works with ligament patients will know how far a patient can safely be pushed; more often than not, we have found that many rehab centers don't expect enough from these patients, which can dramatically slow the patient's recovery.

Rehabilitation for ligament reconstruction is typically broken down into four phases.

Phase 1

Getting out of bed the first day wasn't that bad—the noninjured leg moved fine. The other one just sort of sat there like it was dead. I had to pick it up by the brace and put it on the floor.

ACL patient

Very often, ACL rehabilitation is a fight against time. After an ACL reconstruction, the knee can get very stiff, which can quickly lead to immobility. Movement can be painful and difficult. Patients are encouraged to use the CPM machine while in the hospital and also at home.

In the initial period after surgery (from week 1 to 3) the primary goal is to gain full range of motion (at least 0 to 120 degrees flexion) within 3 to 4 weeks and to relearn the normal gait cycles. Every 1 to 2 days, you should strive to increase 10 degrees of motion. Full weight bearing with crutches is encouraged immediately until you feel secure (usually by 3 weeks) at which point the crutches are no longer used. During this time, you are encouraged to do straight leg-raising exercises and active flexion and extension (bending and straightening).

You are encouraged to walk with the aid of crutches. Movement can be painful, and you may want to take an analgesic before physical therapy. This may be fine, but talk to your doctor and physical therapist before doing so. If you take painkillers before therapy, there is a risk that you may harm a structure if you push too hard. Remember, your ultimate goal is pain-free, drug-free living, and that can only be achieved through proper exercise.

Phase 2. The fourth week through about the ninth week is a critical period because the reconstructed ligament begins to weaken, which is part of the healing process. By the fifth or sixth week, you begin resistive exercises—trying to strengthen the stabilizing muscles around the knee. This can be accomplished by a technique called *contract relax;* for example, you attempt isometrically to contract or tense up a muscle for 5 to 6 seconds and then stretch the same muscle. Functional activities are also begun, such as stair climbing and single leg support. You usually discard the brace as soon as you are comfortable with walking without it. You may then wear a knee sleeve, which is usually a neoprene-type soft brace with a hole for the kneecap.

Phase 3. Depending on your progress, between 12 to 13 weeks and about 4 months, the emphasis shifts from strengthening to functional training. Exercises should be specifically geared to your activities; for example, if you want to return to playing tennis or basketball, you will be given exercises that can help you learn how to cut or pivot.

Phase 4. Between 4 and 5 months postsurgery, the final phase of recovery is geared to returning you to normal activity. Strength training continues; we periodically check the ligament for strength and endurance using special machines and functional tests. For example, KT 2000 testing is a pain-free test that measures forward and backward movement of the tibia relative to the femur.

For specific exercises for ligament rehabilitation, see page 171.

Fractures

Your skeleton is an amazing structure. It is lightweight enough to allow for easy movement, yet powerful enough to withstand tremendous force. Although bones are rigid, they are also flexible and bend when outside force is applied to them.

Every time you run or jump, the bones that make up your knee joint "give" ever so slightly and then return to their normal shape. However, as durable as bones may be, if the force exerted on them becomes too great, the bones will break. In addition, bones may be weakened by diseases such as osteoporosis, which can cause thin, brittle bones that are more prone to injury.

A fracture is an actual break in a bone; there are several kinds of fractures, some serious, some not. Some may mend on their own within a few weeks; some may require major surgery and take months of healing.

Stress Fractures

"I played a lot of tennis over the weekend, and I woke up Monday morning and my knee was killing me. I limped around for a week or so, and then I felt a lot better." When I hear this kind of complaint from a patient who otherwise checks out to be completely normal, I immediately consider the possibility that he may have had a stress fracture. A stress fracture is a microscopic crack in the bone's surface. Although it is not a serious injury, it can be a very painful one.

Stress fractures can occur when bones are overworked. If you sliced a piece of bone and looked at it under a high-powered microscope, you would see that bone is a hotbed of activity. Bone cells are constantly engaged in a process called *remodeling*: new bone is being laid down by bone-building cells called *osteoblasts* while old bone is being absorbed by cells called *osteoclasts*. In fact, an adult skeleton turns over every 7 years, and a child's skeleton turns over even more rapidly. Stress fractures can occur when normal force is applied to bone at a time when it is remodeling. Overworked and overstressed, the bone gives way, resulting in microscopic cracks. The only symptom of a stress fracture is pain and tenderness to the touch. Most people have had stress fractures at one time or another and may not have even have realized it. The pain may be here one day and gone the next, and all is forgotten. However, if the pain persists—and sometimes it does—it may warrant an examination by a physician, mostly to rule out other potential problems.

Diagnosis

Physical Examination.   The only positive finding on a physical examination is localized tenderness at the site of the stress fracture. Occasionally, there might be associated swelling. The stress fracture is rarely, if ever, intraarticular (within the joint) but more characteristically on the tibia (shinbone).

An MRI or Bone Scan.   Because it is so small, a stress fracture cannot be detected on plain X rays until the bone begins to heal, and the body lays down a *callus,* a layer of new bone over the crack. A normal X ray may not be able to pick up an early stress fracture, but a bone scan or an MRI will note the increased vascularity, which will have a characteristic pattern for stress fractures.

Treatment

Stress fractures normally heal by the themselves within 3 to 6 weeks. Ice and over-the-counter analgesics can help to relieve pain. Any activity that causes a great deal of discomfort during this healing period should be avoided, otherwise, you can pursue your usual activities.

Complete Fractures

When a bone actually breaks into two or more pieces, it is called a *complete fracture.* A complete fracture can be caused by any type of trauma, including a fall off a bicycle, a car accident, or even a sports injury. Complete fractures are very painful. Some fractures are more serious than others. In a simple or closed fracture, the bone does not break through the skin. However, in an open or compound fracture, bone fragments protrude through the skin, which are more prone to infection in both the wound and the bone. Even in the case of a closed fracture in which the bone does not puncture the skin, the sharp, jagged edges of a severed bone can cut a nerve or slice through a blood vessel, which can lead to serious complications. Therefore, complete bone fractures require immediate medical attention. However, chances are, if you have a serious fracture, you will be in so much pain that no one is going to have to tell you to see a doctor. You will probably not be able to walk on your own and will need to be taken to your physician or nearby emergency room for treatment.

There are several types of complete fractures that may affect the knee bones.

Transverse.   A transverse fracture, which is the most common fracture among adults, occurs when the bone is sliced into two pieces straight across the width of the bone. The ends of the bone may be jagged, and there is often soft-tissue damage.

Comminuted.   In this type of fracture, the bone is smashed into little pieces like a shattered eggshell. A comminuted fracture may occur in a car accident if the knee smashes into the dashboard, and the patella gets broken up into tiny splinters.

Oblique.   In an oblique fracture, the bone is broken on a slant, which is often a result of rotational force.

Spiral.   In a spiral fracture, the break literally spirals around the bone, creating a long, curved fracture.

Is It Displaced or Nondisplaced?

Bone fractures tend to heal themselves in a process that I will explain later, and in most cases, your physician will simply let nature take its course. However, there are times when surgical intervention is necessary. Surgery is almost always required in the case of a displaced fracture when a bone breaks in such a way that even if it mends on its own, its normal strength and shape cannot be restored. If the fractured bone is an integral part of a joint—such as the knee—it can become the weak link in the joint, eventually destroying the anatomy and balance of the joint. For example, many older people fall and fracture their knee in an area called the *tibia plateau,* the location where the articular cartilage sits on the bone. If the injury displaces the tibia plateau by more than a few millimeters, it can throw off the entire alignment of the knee joint and cause severe arthritic changes. Therefore, this kind of injury requires surgical correction to restore the joint.

Diagnosis

Physical Examination.   A fracture about the knee is quite painful and the patient will not move the knee very much, if at all. There will usually be immediate swelling and tenderness at the site of fracture. Within a few hours, the area will be black and blue.

An X-ray.   Complete bone fractures can be diagnosed by X ray, which will show the location of the fracture and the type of break.

Computerized Axial Tomographic Scanning (CAT Scan). A CAT scan is a regular X ray that transects the bone into serial sections, either from front to back or from the side. It is sometimes used to help assess the depth of a subtle fracture.

Treatment

If the fracture is stable, that is, if the broken bones can firmly reattach, surgery is not required. The more surface area involved in the break, the more likely the fracture is stable. For example, a long spiral fracture is usually more stable than a transverse fracture that neatly splits the bone in two and has very little surface area. If the fracture is stable, the leg is casted until it mends—a so-called closed reduction procedure. Closed reduction, which requires no incision, is often performed under general anesthesia. In this procedure, the bones are put back in their normal position and held in place by a cast. When the fracture is healed, the cast is removed. An experienced knee surgeon can usually predict whether a closed reduction will be successful prior to surgery.

If, however, the fracture is unstable, that is, if the bones cannot reattach without becoming wobbly—as in the case of a transverse fracture—a surgical procedure called *open reduction and internal fixation* may be required. If an open reduction is necessary, it will require an appropriate incision and internal fixation of the fracture fragment with hardware, plates, screws, and, possibly, rods. The recovery time from the surgery depends on the injury and individual. The principle of rehabilitation is to allow knee joint motion as early as possible while protecting the fracture from excessive weight-bearing stress. The rehabilitation program varies depending on the type of injury.

Nondisplaced Fractures

Bone has an amazing capacity to heal itself. After a bone breaks, the process of building new bone begins. Blood rushes to the wounded area, forming a fracture hematoma, or mass of blood that protects the injury. New, immature bone cells begin to form around the injury. In a process that can take between 6 weeks and 6 months, the immature bone cells mature and develop into solid bone, and the broken bones eventually knit back together.

At one time, we used to automatically put the injured limb in a cast to prevent overstressing the fracture while it heals. However, we have since learned that complete immobilization can seriously weaken the leg muscles; therefore, we now try to stress-relieve the wounded area with crutches and a functional cast made of fiberglass that allows for some movement. By doing this, we can prevent weight from being put on the broken bone, but the knee can still have some range of motion, which will prevent the muscles from atrophying.

Displaced Fractures

Displaced fractures are surgical emergencies that can be treated by either closed reduction or open reduction, depending on the type of injury.

Related Injuries

Bone Bruise

A bruise can occur when a force is exerted to tissue around the bone that actually breaks microscopic blood vessels. Instead of flowing through its normal pipeline, the blood spills out, staining the bone and causing inflammation.

Diagnosis.   Although a bone bruise can be painful, it is not nearly as painful as a serious fracture, and you will be able to move your knee through a normal range of motion. An MRI will show a bone bruise.

Treatment.   The bleeding usually stops within a short period of time, and the bone bruise heals on its own. Ice will reduce the inflammation.

Growth Epiphyseal Plate Fractures

A fracture in a child can be a cause for concern if it occurs on an area of bone that is still growing—the so-called growth epiphyseal plate. Epiphyseal fractures are very worrisome, because should they not heal correctly, both the angular alignment of the leg and its overall length will be adversely affected.

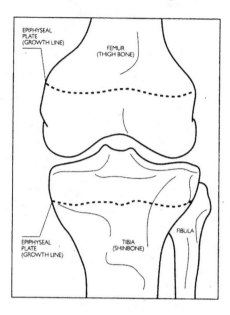

If the growth plate is symmetrically (medially and laterally) injured, there is a possibility that the injured leg will not grow as long as the uninjured leg. If the injury is asymmetric (only on one side of the leg), then the uninjured side will continue to grow while the injured side won't, which could result in an angular deformity. The younger the child, the more potential for growth disturbance. Growth epiphyseal plate fractures are treated the same as other fractures.

Patellar Tendinitis

Tendons are strong, fibrous bands that connect muscle to bone. *Tendinitis* is the inflammation of a tendon. What is commonly known as the patellar tendon is actually a ligament because it connects the patella, or kneecap, to the tibia. However, for simplicity's sake, I will also refer to the patellar ligament as the patellar tendon.

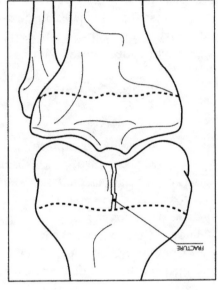

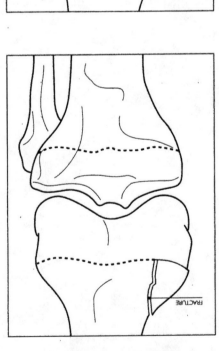

FRACTURE

FRACTURE

Both tendons and ligaments are very complex structures; they consist of millions of tiny microscopic fibers or fibrils. When a tendon or ligament is overused, it doesn't tear in the classic sense, rather it becomes stretched out like a worn-out rubber band. If you looked at the ligament or tendon under a high-powered microscope, you would see that there are microscopic tears in the tiny fibrils. If you tear enough of these fibrils, the area will become inflamed and you will feel sore. "Jumper's knee" is a form of tendinitis that afflicts basketball players. Too much of almost anything that puts pressure on the knee—dancing, cycling, or even hiking—can also cause tendinitis.

Diagnosis

This is one you can diagnose yourself: if you have patellar tendinitis, you will have localized tenderness at the point of insertion where the tendon meets the bone. You will probably feel some discomfort if you try to run or jog.

Treatment

Treating tendinitis is a delicate balance between giving the area time to heal and simultaneously strengthening the muscles that support the leg. If you are initially in a great deal of discomfort, ice, rest, and elevation of the area may relieve your symptoms. Over-the-counter analgesics such as aspirin or ibuprofen may help relieve some of the inflammation.

As soon as possible, you should begin doing some gentle leg exercises; if you don't exercise the muscles, they will quickly begin to weaken, which will ultimately only make matters worse. Don't push yourself to extreme discomfort; do such simple but effective exercises as gently extending and flexing your leg in warm water or using a stationary bike at low tension. Avoid doing any vigorous quadriceps-strengthening exercises that might pull on the area. When the pain subsides, you should gradually return to your normal exercise routine. Tendinitis is not a serious problem and will usually heal on its own. If the discomfort persists for more than 3 weeks and you don't see a trend for the better, call your physician.

Quadriceps Tendon Rupture

You're walking down a flight of stairs, you trip, and your quadriceps muscles contract violently, pulling on the tendon in an attempt to break the fall. The excessive force on the tendon can result in a quadriceps tendon rupture or tear. A quadriceps tendon rupture is a fairly common injury among people past fifty. It is primarily due to a weakening of the tendon caused by a reduction in blood supply to the lower extremities.

Very often, patients with a quadriceps tendon rupture or patellar tendon rupture had been given steroid injections into their tendons when they were younger. This practice is no longer considered safe: we now know that steroid injections into tendons can predispose you to a latent rupture and should not be used.

Diagnosis

A complete quadriceps tendon rupture is quite painful, and it is extremely difficult to move the leg. In fact, you will not be able to bend, extend, or lift your injured leg from either a lying down or sitting position. The knee will swell almost immediately after the injury.

On physical examination, the physician can usually feel a defect in the tendon at the site of the tear.

In some cases, the tendon may rupture only partially. Although the injury is painful, you may still be able weakly to lift and extend the leg.

In the case of a ruptured quadriceps tendon, an X ray of the knee will show the patella in a somewhat lower position (a few millimeters) on the knee than normal.

If the physician suspects that the rupture is only a partial one, she may order an MRI to confirm the diagnosis.

Treatment

A complete rupture will require open-knee surgery as soon as possible. The surgeon must first even up the two ripped ends of the tendon, reattach them, and suture the repaired tendon back in place. After surgery, the leg must be casted for anywhere from 3 to 6 weeks.

A partial tear can be casted without surgery. Both injuries will require a substantial rehabilitation program.

Rehabilitation

The goal of rehabilitation is to restore motion without disrupting the reconstructed tendon. The exercises are similar to those of a ligament rehabilitation program but are less aggressive and will vary widely from patient to patient. Once the cast is removed, the initial goal of rehabilitation is to restore range of motion from 0 degrees to 120 degrees of flexion so that you can straighten and flex your knee. After that, you are given exercises designed to build up the strength in the injured leg so that it is equal to the noninjured leg. Although the total rehabilitation can take up to 6 months, nearly all patients will be able to return to their preinjury levels of sports participation.

Patellar Tendon Rupture

You're playing basketball, you come down from a rebound, and suddenly you're in terrible pain. Your knee swells up, and you can't straighten your leg. This is the typical scenario of a patellar tendon rupture, an injury that most often affects people in their forties while they are engaging in physical activity, although in more rare cases, it could also be caused by another type of injury, such as a fall.

In some cases, the tendon may only be partially ruptured, which is painful but not as serious as a complete rupture.

Diagnosis

Similar to a quadriceps tendon rupture, patients with a patellar tendon rupture will not be able to straighten their injured leg. In addition, they will be in a great deal of pain.

On an X ray, the patella will appear in a somewhat higher position (a few millimeters higher) on the knee than normal.

An MRI can determine if the rupture is complete or partial.

Treatment

A complete rupture must be surgically repaired with open-knee surgery. The tendon ends must be cleaned, reattached, and sutured back to the patella or tibia, depending on the location of the tear. You will then be casted for anywhere from 3 to 6 weeks, and once the cast is removed, you will begin exercises to restore your full range of motion. Leg strengthening exercises are also essential to help build up strength in the injured leg so that it is equal to the noninjured leg.

Bursitis

Bursa are small, fluid-filled sacs located around the knee and other joints throughout the body. The primary purpose of bursa is to lubricate the joint and reduce friction. Bursitis can occur when bursa become irritated from an injury such as banging the knee or chronic wear and tear. For example, a well-known problem related to overuse called "housemaid's knee" is actually caused by the inflammation of the prepatellar bursa, the sac lying in front of the kneecap. Although the affected knee can swell up and look really terrible, the condition is not serious and is rarely painful.

Diagnosis

Bursitis of the knee is diagnosed by physical examination. There is a noticeable swelling on top of the patella.

Treatment

In most cases, you don't need to see a physician for bursitis of the knee. Simply ice the affected area to reduce inflammation, and then forget about it. In the majority of cases, the excess fluid will be reabsorbed into the body. In rare instances, if someone finds that the fluid buildup is particularly uncomfortable, the physician may insert a needle into the bump to aspirate the fluid. However, this procedure can lead to infection and scarring, and I rarely recommend it.

Synovial Plicae

In the womb, an embryo has a very specific way of developing, and many of the structures that are vital during the early life of an embryo are not necessary as the fetus becomes more mature. These structures are called *embryological remnants,* and that is what synovial plicae are. During the first 2 months of an embryo's life, the knee is composed of three synovial compartments separated by thin walls or fibrous bands of tissue called *plicae.* However, by the fourth month of fetal life, the knee develops into one compartment, and the plicae should rupture or disappear. However, in about 70 percent of the population, a portion, if not all, of the plicae remains in the knee joint. In rare cases, plicae, which are like tiny rubber bands, can be very troublesome. At times, plicae can get caught between the kneecap and the femur, causing pain and discomfort. Plicae can also abraid the surface of articular cartilage, which not only can destroy the cartilage, but can also cause a snapping sensation in the knee, which can be quite uncomfortable.

Diagnosis

Symptomatic plicae is a diagnosis of exclusion: if nothing else is wrong, there is a possibility that the problem is caused by synovial plicae. Plicae can only be seen through an arthroscope, and in my opinion, the belief that plicae are to blame for knee problems is probably the cause of many an unnecessary arthroscopy. If you are in pain for no apparent reason, more likely it is caused by a malaligned kneecap than plicae. Before arthroscopy is undertaken to check for plicae problems, all other possibilities should be considered first. In addition, you should undergo a well-supervised exercise strengthening program before looking for potential plicae problems. (I stress well supervised because if someone is doing exercises inappropriately, it could actually be causing their knee pain.) If everything else fails, then plicae should be considered as a source of the pain.

Treatment

In cases where plicae bands are actually causing real problems, your surgeon can simply cut them out during an arthroscopy, finishing the job that nature started. However, it's often difficult to determine whether cutting plicae is really going to make a significant difference. Time will tell. If you feel better within 6 to 8 months, you know that the plicae were the source of the trouble.

Arthritis

Arthritis—the inflammation of a joint—can be caused by a multitude of factors ranging from inflammatory conditions, such as rheumatoid arthritis and lupus, to osteoarthritis, which is caused by the degeneration of the joint caused by wear and tear.

The end result of an arthritic condition is the destruction of *articular cartilage* (also known as *hyaline cartilage*), the unique substance that lines the joints, preventing the bone endings from rubbing together. The smooth, thin, but resilient lining of articular cartilage allows the joints to move in a fluid fashion and protects bone from excessive force or pressure. As the articular cartilage gets worn down, the bones become more exposed, resulting in pain, stiffness, and swelling in the joints.

Some forms of arthritis are very mild and may be limited to an occasional twinge on a rainy day. But in some cases, arthritis can progressively destroy a joint, causing great pain and severely limiting movement.

Arthritis can be caused by more than 100 different conditions, ranging from bone tumors to gout (a condition characterized by deposits of uric acid crystals in the joint) to a glitch in the immune system that can trigger a disease such as systemic lupus erythematosus. Arthritic symptoms can even be caused by Lyme disease, which is spread by a spirochete (a spiral-shaped organism) and transmitted by ticks. Any injury to the articular cartilage, such as a bad fall or a direct blow to a joint, can also promote arthritic changes as can an injury to a ligament that may disrupt the normal alignment of the knee.

There are two forms of arthritis that are most common—osteoarthritis and rheumatoid arthritis—and these are the ones that I see most often in my practice. Although they often have the same end result—the destruction of joints—they are actually quite different.

Osteoarthritis

Some 16 million Americans, many of them elderly, have osteoarthritis (OA), also known as wear and tear or degenerative arthritis. (This is not to be confused with osteoporosis, a common condition caused by the demineralization of bones. See page 155.) Studies of X rays show that more than 75 percent of all people over fifty-five have some form of OA, although some may not experience symptoms. OA can strike any joint, but it is most likely to affect the large weight-bearing joints of the lower limbs, such as the knees. Symptoms of OA include morning stiffness that usually disappears within a half hour or so after rising and pain (with or without inflammation).

As the articular cartilage is worn away, the *condyles,* the knobby exposed ends of the femur and tibia, become hard and shiny. The joint space narrows, and in the late stages of this process, the joint lays down small spurs of bone called *osteophytes.* The osteophytes provide some stability by filling in the empty space, but they can also make the knee feel stiff. The synovial membranes—the membranes lining the joint—become thickened and secrete fluid rich in proteolytic enzymes. Although initially protective, this fluid can eventually be destructive, eating away at the articular cartilage. As the arthritis progresses, bone is literally rubbing against bone. This can throw off the normal alignment of the knee, resulting in deformities such as knock-knees or bowlegs.

Diagnosis

Physical Examination. Patients with OA often have pain and limited range of motion in one or both knees. An examination of your knee may reveal telltale osteophytes or bone spurs and will also reveal any angular deformities, such as bowlegs or knock-knees.

An X Ray. A conventional X ray (it must be done in a standing position so the joint is compressed) will show the narrowed spaces in the joint due to the loss of articular cartilage as well as any osteophytes. Very often, non–knee surgeons will just order supine X rays. These are a waste of money for an arthritic population.

Treatment

There is no cure for arthritis; as of now, there is no way to restore lost articular cartilage. Nor do we know how to stop this disease from progressing. However, there are ways to reduce pain with medications such as aspirin, ibuprofin, naproxen, or other NSAIDs (see page 111).

More importantly, a good exercise rehabilitation program can improve mobility and decrease discomfort. At the end of this chapter, I have included an exercise program designed for people with degenerative arthritis. In advanced cases, a surgical procedure known as an *osteotomy,* or a total knee replacement, may be required.

Weight Loss. Very often, if you are overweight, weight loss can reduce the pressure on the knee joint and may relieve symptoms. In a recent study that appeared in *The Annals of Internal Medicine,* researchers examined whether weight loss would significantly reduce the risk of developing knee OA in overweight women. Based on their study, they found that a modest weight loss of about 5.1 kilograms (about 2.5 pounds) over the 10 years before assessment reduced the odds of developing knee OA by 50 percent. The researchers also noted that weight change after age forty greatly affected the risk of developing knee OA.

Alternative Remedies.   There are many other popular remedies that are used to treat arthritis. Natural food stores are filled with so-called arthritis remedies ranging from herbs such as wild yam, evening primrose oil, and propolis (a substance derived from bee pollen) to boswellin cream, an ointment made from the *Boswellia serrata* plant, which is used in traditional Indian medicine and is reputed to soothe stiff joints. There have been few serious scientific studies to investigate these alternative treatments, and most of those that have been performed have been done outside of the United States. Nevertheless, many patients claim that some of these folk remedies help to relieve their symptoms.

Keep in mind that medicine is not an exact science, and even though we may not understand why, it's possible that some people may actually get relief from some of these remedies. In some cases, these remedies may simply be placebos, but in other cases, these substances may work in ways that we don't understand. When patients ask me if they should try some of these unproven remedies, I often tell them that they may not hurt, and in fact, some may actually be helpful. However, when it comes to a chronic disease such as arthritis, which can cause a great deal of misery for so many people, there is also a great deal of fraud and false claims. Be wary of parting too easily with your money or experimenting with questionable therapies that could cause harm. In particular, be wary of using drugs that are sold overseas but are not approved for use in the United States. Don't believe advertisements that appear in the back of magazines or tabloids—there is no wonder drug for arthritis.

Arthroscopy. If conventional therapies fail to relieve the pain or improve mobility, your surgeon may perform an arthroscopy to remove any debris such as pieces of articular cartilage that are floating around the joint, which could cause inflammation, or to smooth out any rough edges that could also be causing a synovial or inflammatory response. About 75 percent of all patients will find short-term symptomatic relief from this procedure.

Surgery. If all else fails, the surgeon will consider realigning the joint (an osteotomy) or a total knee replacement.

Rheumatoid Arthritis

About 2.1 million Americans have rheumatoid arthritis (RA), which afflicts three times as many women as men. RA is a chronic inflammatory disease that occurs when the body's immune system is thrown out of whack and begins to attack its own tissue. The synovial lining of the joint becomes inflamed, and the synovial fluid begins to invade the rest of the joint, destroying the articular cartilage down to the bone and then eventually destroying the bone. RA usually first appears in the joints of the fingers and spreads to the wrists, knuckles, and knees. It can also present in the knee first. The initial symptoms include swelling, warmth, and redness in one or more joints. In more serious cases, RA can also cause extreme fatigue, fever, weight loss, and a susceptibility to infection. As it progresses, RA not only wreaks havoc on joints, but can destroy soft tissue (such as ligaments and tendons) and damage to the coverings of the heart, lungs, eyes, and other organs. In acute cases, soft-tissue nodules may appear, usually on the fingers, which are often accompanied by fever and general malaise.

No one knows what causes RA; however, many researchers believe that it is triggered by an unidentified virus that somehow alters the immune system.

Unlike OA, RA tends to be polyarticular, which means that it often affects two joints symmetrically. (There is one exception: in children, RA tends to strike one joint, especially the knee.) In addition, morning stiffness from RA tends to last longer than stiffness from OA and may affect the muscles as well as the joints.

Early diagnosis of RA is important; researchers have recently learned that RA can be most destructive to joints in its earliest stages. Although RA can't be cured, some treatments may help to keep the disease at bay, thus preventing the rapid destruction of joints.

Anyone with RA should be treated by a rheumatologist, a specialist in connective tissue disease who is well versed with the many drugs and therapies for RA and is trained to deal with the day-to-day management of this chronic disease. However, an orthopedist may be consulted if an orthopedic problem arises, for example, if the joint destruction progresses to the point where the patient requires surgery.

Diagnosis

Based on the American Rheumatism Association's 1987 revised criteria for the classification of RA, you must have four of seven of the following criteria to be diagnosed with RA.

- Morning stiffness.
- Arthritis of three or more joint areas.
- Arthritis of hand joints.
- Rheumatoid nodules.
- Serum rheumatoid factor.
- Radiographic changes (changes apparent in an X ray).

During the physical examination, your physician will look for these and other changes that could pinpoint the diagnosis. Upon examination, he may see signs of swelling and inflammation or the soft-tissue nodules that often appear in acute cases. Your medical history is also important; you may be experiencing other symptoms that could point to a diagnosis of

RA. The family medical history is also relevant, because RA often runs in families.

A standing X ray will show the narrowing of the joint spaces due to the erosion of articular cartilage or destruction to the bone itself. Changes due to RA are different than those due to OA.

There are several blood tests that may also point to a diagnosis of RA:

Complete Blood Count.   Blood counts can tell a great deal about overall health. In the case of an inflammatory disease such as RA, the white blood cell count is often elevated. In addition, many patients have low levels of red blood cells, which is called anemia of chronic disease.

Rheumatoid Factor.   About 75 percent of all patients with RA will test positive for antibodies called *rheumatoid factor* in their blood.

Sedimentation Rate (Erythrocyte Sedimentation Rate, or ESR). People who have active inflammation will have an elevated ESR. However, there are many conditions, including tumors and other autoimmune diseases, that can elevate the ESR.

Synovial Fluid Analysis.   In this test, a small amount of synovial fluid is aspirated from the joint and analyzed in a laboratory. In RA, the fluid will show specific changes due to inflammation: the glucose level may drop, and the white cell count will rise.

Treatment

NSAIDs.   In about 50 percent of all cases, the symptoms are mild enough to be managed by over-the-counter or prescription NSAIDs such as aspirin, ibuprofen, and naproxen.

Exercise.   At one time, patients with RA were told to refrain from strenuous exercise; we now know that many people with this disease will actually benefit from vigorous workouts. In addition to maintaining flexibility and muscle tone, exercise can also reduce fatigue and the feelings of helplessness often associated with RA. However, joint-sparing exercise, such as swimming, water exercises in a heated pool, cycling, and working out on a cross-country ski machine, is preferable to weight-bearing exercise that may further weaken susceptible joints. If you have RA, consult your physician or physical therapist about which exercise regime is right for you. In addition, the Arthritis Foundation offers some excellent information on safe exercise for arthritis patients.

Stronger Drugs.   At one time, most physicians took a wait-and-see approach with the treatment of RA. Typically, they began with the milder NSAIDs and waited—sometimes years—to progress to stronger drugs as they were needed. Today, however, for more severe cases, doctors are now prescribing stronger medications early on in the hopes of halting the inflammatory process before it can inflict its damage upon the affected joints. Although NSAIDs may still be the first line of defense against RA, if the patient doesn't improve within a few months, many physicians will switch therapies. For example, the powerful anticancer drug methotrexate (Rheumatrex) may now be prescribed after the initial diagnosis of RA. Unlike other medications to treat RA that can take months to be effective, methotrexate begins to work within a few weeks. Studies have shown that methotrexate has milder side effects than many other anticancer drugs; however, there are some potentially dangerous complications, including a slightly increased risk of liver damage. (According to one recent study, the risk of developing serious liver disease due to methotrexate is about 1 in 1,000 at 5 years of use.) Anyone on this drug must be monitored closely by her physician but not as closely as we once thought. In the past, patients on this drug were given routine liver biopsies, but new guidelines recommend that patients on methotrexate undergo blood tests every 4 to 8 weeks to check for any irregularity in liver enzymes. Other medications given for RA include hydroxychloroquine sulfate, an antimalarial drug, which has few side effects, and injectable gold salts (gold sodium thiomalate or aurothioglucose). In addition, steroids such as prednisone or other drugs that suppress the immune system, such as azathioprine, may be prescribed, but they can leave the patient vulnerable to infection and result in severe anemia. Any patients on these drugs should be closely monitored by their physicians. (Long-term use of steroids is not advisable: these drugs can cause the destruction of bone as well as a slew of other problems.)

Arthroscopy. If conventional therapies fail to relieve the pain or improve mobility, your surgeon may perform an arthroscopy to remove any debris, such as pieces of articular cartilage, that are floating around the joint, which could cause inflammation, or to smooth out any rough edges that could also be causing a synovial or inflammatory response. About 75 percent of all patients will find short-term symptomatic relief from this procedure. In some cases, a synovectomy, the removal of the synovium, may be necessary and can be performed arthroscopically.

Surgery.   If all else fails, the surgeon will consider realigning the joint (osteotomy) or a total knee replacement. (For a full explanation of osteotomy and total knee replacement, see page 129.)

Rehabilitation Training for OA

The primary goals of an exercise program for OA are to maximize the range of motion, strengthen the extensor mechanism and leg flexion (the quadriceps muscles and hamstrings), and reduce pain. Numerous studies confirm that strength training can reduce the pain of arthritis by turning nearby muscles into shock absorbers, reducing the force exerted on the joint. Exercise also helps to improve mobility and to prevent excessive weight gain, which can also promote arthritis.

However, some forms of exercise—particularly those that place excessive force on the knee joints—may hurt more than they may help. Exercises that increase the force through the knee in an axial (up/down) fashion, such as jumping, jogging, and running, should be avoided. Joint-sparing exercise, such as swimming, bicycling, and any exercises done in a warm-water pool, are all excellent ways to maintain mobility without further damaging your knee joints. (For exercises for OA, turn to page 171.)

CHAPTER 4

Coping with Knee Pain

Whether you're dealing with the pain of an acute injury or the nagging ache and discomfort typical of a chronic problem such as arthritis, the methods are similar with a few important exceptions. This chapter explains everything you need to know to deal with both kinds of pain.

Ice

After an acute injury, an ice pack applied directly to the injured area can reduce both pain and swelling. Use ice for 15-minute intervals and repeat as needed. Theoretically, ice causes a vasoconstriction (the localized blood flow is decreased due to a contraction of the vessels as a response to cold), which simultaneously diminishes the inflammatory process. Do not apply heat to a fresh injury; it will swell and may actually heighten the pain.

Heat

Heat tends to stimulate the blood supply to the joint. It's somewhat idiosyncratic in application. Some patients really like it, others don't. Don't use it right after activities, but try it before exercise to help warm up.

Rubs and Ointments

The shelves of pharmacies and natural food stores are packed with creams and lotions designed to reduce joint pain and inflammation due to arthritis. There are several popular creams that contain eucalyptus oil, which increases the blood flow to the area, thus producing a feeling of warmth. Capsaicin cream, which is made from a compound extracted from chili peppers, has also been found to offer temporary relief for arthritis. Similar to eucalyptus, it works by irritating the skin, promoting blood flow and creating a sensation of warmth. Many practitioners of alternative medicine swear by boswellin cream, an ointment made from the *Boswellia serrata* plant that is used in traditional Indian medicine to soothe stiff joints. Since the 1980s, dimethyl sulfoxide (DMSO) has been used externally to treat pain and arthritis. DMSO comes in liquid, cream, and roll-on. DMSO has one unpleasant side effect: it can result in garlic-breath.

These creams may work well for some people but not others; there's no harm in trying to see if one may work for you. They are relatively safe, but there is a potential risk of developing a skin irritation. If you do get a rash, discontinue use.

Acetaminophen

Marketed under such names as Tylenol, Panedol, and Datril, acetaminophen is basically an analgesic that can relieve muscle pain. However, it is not an anti-inflammatory and does little for arthritis or to reduce swelling due to an injury.

Nonsteroidal Anti-inflammatory Drugs (NSAIDs)

The term *NSAIDs* refers to a class of drugs that is commonly used to treat pain and inflammation. There are many different types of NSAIDs, ranging from simple aspirin to ibuprofin (Advil and Motrin) to naproxen (Naprosyn). Many NSAIDs are sold over the counter, although many of the less-well-known ones are sold by prescription. There are too many NSAIDs on the market to cite by name, and each month, new NSAIDs are introduced by pharmaceutical companies.

Although they are all somewhat different in action, all NSAIDs work to alleviate the inflammatory process. Most of the drugs inhibit the inflammatory process, often blocking substances, such as prostaglandins, that are mediators of the inflammatory process. Each drug works on a different level of the inflammatory cycle. Unfortunately, none of these drugs can prevent the real cause of the inflammation—in other words, they are treatments and not cures. As a result, over time, NSAIDs can become ineffective. Very often, a drug will work well for up to a year, and then its positive effect will wear off. What probably happens is the body simply works around the drug: the inflammatory cycle is a cascade of events that consists of several levels. If the drug blocks the inflammatory cycle at one level in the inflammatory cycle, the inflammation simply continues on another. Switching to another NSAID may help.

For an acute injury, NSAIDs can be used for 7 to 10 days, taken every 3 to 4 hours as needed. Dosage varies with each drug. Generally, it takes anywhere from 12 to 36 hours to get a high-enough blood level of the drug to have a noticeable effect.

The effects of NSAIDs are highly individualistic: some people may find one type of NSAID better than another.

NSAIDs can have significant side effects, notably gastrointestinal bleeding, gastric upset, and stomach bleeding, and may even promote ulcers. The gastric problems caused by NSAIDs are due to its antiprostaglandin effect: although prostaglandins can cause inflammation in other parts of the body, they help to protect the stomach lining against irritation.

Many arthritic patients rely on NSAIDs to control pain. NSAIDs should not be taken on a long-term basis unless it is done under a doctor's supervision, preferably a rheumatologist who is skilled in tailoring these medications to patients. When the drug is initially prescribed, you should be closely monitored for signs of adverse reaction. Blood chemistry should be checked every month for up to 3 months to monitor liver and renal function, which can be impaired by these drugs. If all is well, you should then be rechecked at 6 months. If you show no sign of any problem after that, the blood can be checked every year.

All patients taking NSAIDs should be aware of the warning signs of potential trouble, which include headache, blood in the stool, bloating, and just not feeling right. Frankly, given the possible side effects that can be caused by these drugs, I have serious reservations about keeping patients on these medicines long term. If you are taking an NSAID for a long period of time, you should discuss possible alternatives with your physician. If the pain is being caused by a mechanical problem, such as the formation of debris in the joint, a minor arthroscopic surgery could be performed to remove the inflammation. Although this is not a permanent solution, it can offer relief for up to 2 years. Sometimes a good exercise strengthening program may help to reduce the need for pain medication. In some cases, if the pain is too debilitating, a total knee replacement should be considered.

Corticosteroids

Corticosteroids are synthetic versions of cortisone, a hormone produced by the adrenal glands. Although cortisone is normally present in the body, in high doses, it can have a therapeutic effect. Cortisone can be taken orally or, in the case of joint pain, can be injected directly into the joint. Oral steroids should only be used by people with problems such as rheumatoid arthritis and lupus under the close supervision of their physicians. Although oral cortisone can relieve pain, it also suppresses the immune system, which can leave you more vulnerable to infection. It can also raise blood pressure, increase cholesterol, and promote osteoporosis—the thinning of the bones and avascular necrosis—or bone death.

In some cases, if you are in a great deal of pain and NSAIDs are ineffective, a physician may give a cortisone injection. There are many potentially dangerous side effects to cortisone shots, and I feel they should be avoided if possible. An occasional cortisone shot does offer relief from pain, but the effect is temporary. It does not cure the problem; it merely masks the discomfort. In addition, in high or repetitive doses, cortisone may actually promote the destruction of the joint by destroying the articular cartilage and the tendons. Thus, cortisone shots should be few and far between; no more than one every 6 months for a maximum of no more than two or three total. You are better off being maintained on oral steroids (under the care of a rheumatologist) or other NSAIDs.

Intraarticular cortisone shots should never be used on children or teenagers unless they suffer from an inflammatory arthritis and are being closely monitored by a rheumatologist.

CHAPTER 5

Preparing for Surgery

Get as much information as possible because your life changes after surgery. It's not just a matter of your doctor going in there and repairing what he has to repair. You have to constantly work at it too. Just coming to rehab three times a week disrupts your normal routine, and after that, you have to continue to exercise for the rest of your life or you'll have another problem.

Patient after meniscal repair

If you are a candidate for knee surgery—whether it is an arthroscopy for arthritis or a ligament repair or a total knee replacement—you should be well informed about your impending procedure and should fully understand both the risks and benefits. In addition, you need to understand that you are a major player in your own health care, and the decisions that you make prior to surgery and the role you play in your own recovery can be every bit as important as the surgical procedure itself. This chapter will help you to be a better-prepared, better-informed patient.

Choosing Your Doctor

Orthopedic surgery should be performed by a board-certified orthopedic surgeon, a physician who, as defined by the American Academy of Orthopedic Surgeons, "specializes in the diagnosis, treatment, rehabilitation and prevention of injuries and diseases of your body's musculoskeletal system." Within the general category of orthopedic surgery, many orthopedists have a subspecialty, that is, they have developed an expertise in treating particular areas, such as the foot, hand, spine, and knee. Subspecialties are usually developed after a fellowship year, which is an additional year after residency. After the individual completes at least a 5-year postmedical school orthopedic residency, he has the option of entering a private practice or doing an extra year of training in a specific area. Theoretically, any board-certified surgeon can perform any type of orthopedic surgery, however, those of us who do surgery recognize that the kind of highly technical procedures that are routinely done today are best performed by those who are subspecialty trained. In other words, if you're having surgery on your hip, you want to be operated on by a surgeon who does a lot of hip operations, and if you're having surgery on your knee, you want it done by a surgeon who is primarily a knee surgeon.

Where do you find a good surgeon? There are several places where you can get referrals to competent physicians:

1. Happy patients are good sources of information. If you know someone who has had a successful knee operation, you can ask her for the name of her physician. However, don't take someone else's word for it: talk to the surgeon yourself before making your decision.

2. You can call the county medical society or the department of orthopedic surgery at a local hospital or medical school for a referral.

3. If you want to check whether a surgeon is board certified, you can call the American Board of Orthopaedic Surgery at (919) 929-7103. You must have the complete name of the physician—the last name alone won't do. The American Board will not reveal anything about the surgeon's competency or success rate, but they will tell you whether he has fulfilled his certification requirements and is fully accredited. For a fee of twenty-eight dollars, you can purchase a list of board-certified orthopedic surgeons broken down by state. In some cases, the directory may be found in a medical library at a hospital or medical school.

4. If you want to check the credentials of a particular physician, you can request an AMA physician profile from the American Medical Association in Chicago. The profile will tell you where the physician went to school, where she is licensed to practice medicine, and which, if any, are her specialties. To request a physician profile, write

   American Medical Association
   535 North Dearborn Street
   Chicago, IL 60610

5. There are two professional organizations that will refer you to a qualified subspecialist in your area. Call or write

   The Knee Society
   6300 North River Road
   Rosemont, IL 60018
   (708) 698-1693

   The American Society for Sports Medicine
   6300 North River Road, Suite 200
   Rosemont, IL 60018
   (708) 292-4900

6. In the reference section of most libraries, there are physician directories compiled by county medical societies and the AMA. Ask your librarian for help.

Don't assume that someone who bills himself as a sports medicine specialist is automatically the best knee surgeon, nor should you assume that if you have a sports injury, a surgeon who specializes in the treatment of arthritis is not competent to do your surgery. Within the past few years, there has been a merger between these two specialties, and we are beginning to see the emergence of knee specialists who handle both kinds of patients. Labels no longer mean anything: one surgeon may be just as good as the other. How do you know if an orthopedic surgeon is a competent knee surgeon? There are several ways to find out. First, check out her credentials. Second, ask the surgeon if she is subspecialty trained as a knee surgeon or if she is a member of the Knee Society or any other subspecialty society. And most importantly, ask the surgeon specifically about how many procedures like yours she performs each year. Although it's hard to give a specific number, you definitely don't want to be operated on by someone who does only four total knees a year or four anterior cruciate ligament reconstructions. I would, however, feel comfortable with a surgeon who does anywhere between twenty-five and fifty procedures a year.

Once you've established that the surgeon is experienced in your procedure, how can you tell if she is a good surgeon? This is a bit trickier to find out but not impossible. Don't be afraid to ask questions: a good surgeon will not be offended by your inquiries or reluctant to answer questions about her background. First, ask the surgeon if she's ever published in any peer review journals—professional journals in which a board of equally qualified physicians review the work of others. If she has, ask to have copies of the articles. Articles and publications in professional journals are an indication that a surgeon is keeping abreast of the latest information and research in her field and has withstood the scrutiny of her peers. However, some surgeons may be excellent at what they do but have no interest in publishing, which doesn't mean that you should dismiss them, but you need to do further checking. Ask to speak to some of her patients who have had your procedure and are in various stages of recovering. This will not only help you to assess the skill of the surgeon, but will give you some idea as to what to expect from the surgery.

Finally, find out about the surgeon's office policy for handling emergencies that may occur after hours. Does she provide a number to call if a problem should arise after you've been released from the hospital? If she's in a group practice, does she refer calls to another physician in her practice, or does she send patients to the nearest emergency room? Although it is rare, complications can arise from knee surgery, and you need to know how the surgeon deals with these problems.

The Second Opinion

Most insurance companies now require a second opinion before they will agree to reimburse the patient for a surgical procedure. There's nothing wrong with getting a second opinion as long as it is from a surgeon who is as qualified as the first. A second opinion from someone who is not a knee specialist is not only useless, but can be quite confusing.

In most cases, surgeons will generally agree on treatment. There are times, however, when surgeons will disagree, and this can be confusing to the patient. Unfortunately, two well-qualified knee surgeons can give two different opinions. Sometimes the second opinion will try to "steal" the patient by telling you what you want to hear. For example, a patient who is clearly terrified of surgery may be easily swayed in favor of a surgeon who downplays surgery and prescribes an exercise program with the caveat that "we'll wait and see what happens." (Sometimes just the reverse is true: a patient is gung ho on surgery because he feels that the surgeon will make him all better with little effort on his part. The overeager surgeon does little to dissuade him of this false notion.) You should have enough knowledge and information to ask pointed questions designed to get at the truth. Some good ones are: Based on past studies, what are my actual chances of recovery without surgery? What can I hope to accomplish from exercise alone? Is there a possibility that my condition can deteriorate further if I postpone surgery? If the surgeon has good statistics to back up her prognosis, then you can feel confident in what she is saying. But if her answers are vague, be suspicious. She may be leading you on—telling you what she thinks you want to hear, not what you need to hear. However, if two equally competent, well-informed surgeons have honestly reached different opinions, a third opinion may be necessary. In this case, you must truly educate yourself to understand all the parameters of your treatment.

Realistic Expectations

Prior to surgery, learn as much about your procedure as possible. Make sure you completely understand the potential benefits and risks of your surgery. Many patients may be reluctant to ask questions because they are afraid of "bothering" their surgeons, they don't want to appear foolish, or their surgeon may appear to be rushed. Although most surgeons are very busy, they should not be too busy to answer important questions. In fact, most welcome questions. From a surgeon's point of view, there is nothing worse than a poorly informed patient who comes in for major knee surgery and thinks that he's going to be back to normal in a few days. When a patient has unrealistic expectations about surgery, he can only be disappointed and frustrated at the outcome, and that can hamper his recovery. Ask your surgeon any questions you may have pertaining to your surgical procedure and recovery, such as potential complications, average rehabilitation time, and when you can resume normal activities such as driving or returning to work. However, there are questions that you should not ask your surgeon. Don't bother her with administrative questions such as inquiries about office hours, insurance forms, and so on. The office staff is there to answer these kinds of questions.

Keep in mind that every patient is different. Even if a friend who had recently had knee surgery was up and running in a month, it doesn't mean that you will be also. Ask your surgeon directly, "Based on my case and my physical condition, what is a realistic recovery time? What should I expect after surgery?" If you know what to expect, you will be better able to prepare for it emotionally and physically.

In addition to asking your surgeon any questions you may have, talk to other patients who have had your procedure. The information and insights that they can provide may be invaluable.

A Presurgical Checklist

- In rare cases, a blood transfusion may be required during surgery. Two weeks before surgery, you should donate blood in the unlikely event that a transfusion will be necessary. Given fears about AIDS, for your own peace of mind, it is preferable to use your own blood. The rule of thumb is, for a single knee replacement, 1 or 2 units of blood is required; for a double knee replacement, 3 or 4 units of blood should be on hand. (Blood is usually not required for procedures other than total knee replacement.)
- A week or two before surgery, you will need to be medically cleared for the operation by your physician.
- If you smoke, you must quit at least 48 hours prior to surgery or risk serious complications. Nicotine, a compound found in tobacco, is broken down by the liver, and its by-products can cause skin problems, which can lead to severe infection and skin loss. Unlike many other joints, the

knee joint is very close to the skin; therefore, it is especially vulnerable to this type of problem.

- If you develop any physical problems prior to surgery, including a fever, infection, or any unusual symptoms, alert your surgeon.
- If you are taking any medication, be sure you tell your internist and your surgeon, and ask specifically whether or not you are to discontinue your medication prior to surgery.
- If you will need assistance at home after surgery, make the appropriate arrangements beforehand. If you don't have any friends or relatives to look after you or if you are responsible for caring for others, talk to the social worker at the hospital about locating the appropriate assistance.
- Make sure you understand the presurgical protocol. In all likelihood, you will be told not to eat or drink after 12 A.M. the night before surgery. If you're having a general anesthetic, your stomach must be empty or you can vomit during anesthesia. If this occurs, you can develop pneumonia.

CHAPTER 6

Picking a Rehabilitation Center

*When I went to the rehab center in my neighborhood,
the first thing I noticed was that they treated every patient the same way. Everyone was doing the same exercises whether they had a hip replacement, a stroke, or a
knee operation. I didn't feel that it was the right thing,
and I wasn't making very much progress, so I went
back to the hospital rehab program even though it
wasn't as convenient.*

A total knee replacement patient

Many knee patients will never come under the surgeon's knife;
in fact, their primary treatment will be a good exercise
strengthening program. In many cases, patients will be referred to a rehabilitation center to work with a physical therapist. However, even if you have surgery, it is no magic bullet.

Depending on the procedure, a patient may spend anywhere from 20 minutes to several hours on the operating
table, but he will be spending several months to a year in rehabilitation for roughly 3 days a week, 45 minutes to an hour at
a time.

Whether or not you have surgery, picking the right rehabilitation center is critical. In my experience, I have found that all

rehabilitation programs are not created equal—some are excellent and give high-quality service and attention to each patient, but as the patient above described, some are merely "rehab" mills where all patients, regardless of their problem, are given the same prescription. Not surprisingly, patients in the poorer-run programs do not fare as well as patients in the better programs. Given your investment in time, money, and hard work, it is essential to find the right rehabilitation program for you. Here are some things you should consider when you are shopping for a rehabilitation center.

Check credentials. The rehabilitation program should be directed by a board-certified physiatrist—a physician who specializes in physical medicine and rehabilitation—who has a special training in knee disorders. Ideally, the physical therapists on staff should be accredited by the American Physical Therapy Association. To further check the reputation of the center, ask to see the physician referral logs. It speaks well of a center if respected orthopedic surgeons feel confident enough in the expertise of the facility to refer their patients.

The center should work with your physician. If you've been referred for rehabilitation, your physical therapist and your physician should stay in close contact to make sure that you are progressing properly. Preferably, you should pick a rehabilitation center that has an established relationship with your physician, knows her approach to treatment, and is willing to adhere to it. Don't go to a rehabilitation center with the expectation that you are being "turned over" to the therapist. Rehabilitation should be based on a prescribed program from your physician.

If you have had an inpatient procedure such as a total knee replacement, an osteotomy, or an anterior cruciate ligament reconstruction, very likely your therapy will begin in the hospital. In fact, at our center, it begins the moment you are rolled out of the operating room and into the recovery room.

Once you leave the hospital, you should continue your therapy at the hospital rehabilitation center if possible. However, if that is not convenient, be sure to choose one that is willing to stay in close communication with your surgeon, who will be monitoring your progress. In some cases, a problem may crop up that may require immediate medical intervention, and your surgeon should be aware of it. In addition, your surgeon needs to know if you are progressing at the expected pace. If you are not making the progress that you should, the surgeon may need to reevaluate your rehab program, or in some cases, further surgery may be required depending on the initial diagnosis.

Experience counts. The rehabilitation center should be experienced in treating your problem. For better or worse, we are living in an era of specialization—one center may be highly skilled in treating stroke patients or shoulder patients but have little expertise with handling knee patients. In addition, a center that treats many older patients who have had knee replacement surgery may not be highly experienced in treating a younger, athletic patient who is recovering from an anterior cruciate ligament reconstruction. How do you know if the center is skilled in your particular problem? Obviously, you need to find a center that has the right training equipment for your problem—your doctor will tell you what to look for—but even that is no assurance that they know how to use it. Further investigation is required. Find out how many patients with problems similar to yours that they have treated within the past year or so. If between one-third and one-half of all patients at the center have your problem or a similar one, that's a good sign.

To assess the level of care, ask if you can speak to some patients. Are they pleased with their treatment? Finally, use your own eyes and ears: look around the center and see what the patients are doing. If all of the patients are performing the same exercises for different problems, something is amiss.

Rehabilitation should be individually tailored to each patient. A good rehabilitation program should be tailored to your needs, condition, and lifestyle. Obviously, a vigorous, athletic person who is anxious to get back on the tennis court is going to have different goals than a sedentary person whose main activities are keeping house and driving to the mall. Your rehabilitation goals should reflect these differences. At the initial meeting with your physiatrist and physical therapist, you want to hear specific information about your needs and your goals and, most importantly, how you will achieve those goals. Simply hearing, "We're going to strengthen your legs and you're going to be fine" is not enough.

A good rehabilitation program should be divided into different phases, and each phase should have a different goal so there is some objective way of measuring your progress. Make sure that the center provides you with a detailed plan before you sign on.

Strong legs are not enough. In addition to strengthening your legs, a good rehab program should address the entire body, including cardiovascular health. Having strong legs does you little good if your aerobic capacity is so poor that you have no endurance. Exercising your heart and lungs is of equal importance.

Supervision. In the first few weeks following surgery, you will need to be closely supervised by a physiatrist and/or physical therapist. After you get the hang of the exercises, you will still need to be monitored but not as closely. Be sure that the center provides intensive supervision in the early phases of your rehabilitation. Avoid places that are clearly overcrowded and understaffed. A good therapist-to-patient ratio is one to two; anything higher could mean that you will not get enough individual attention.

Check out insurance reimbursement. Many but not all insurance companies will pay for some rehabilitative therapy after surgery. Find out what the details of your plan ahead of time. If money is a consideration, as it is for so many people, you may ask the center to try to tailor their plan to accommodate your insurance.

Your future goals. A good exercise rehabilitation program is not just for the duration of your recovery, it is the foundation of a lifetime commitment to exercise and muscle strengthening. Whatever center you choose should be willing to help you plan a permanent exercise regime that you will follow on your own after you are fully recovered.

Once you have selected your rehabilitation center, I recommend that you meet with the therapist before surgery to help you prepare for your operation. For example, if you are going to need to use crutches following surgery, it's a good idea to learn how to use one ahead of time. After your surgery, you will feel tired and a little groggy and may be in pain. You don't need the added pressure of being handed a set of crutches for the first time and being told to walk.

In many cases, it may be advisable to begin your exercise training before surgery. For example, if you are going to need to use a walker or crutches after surgery, you need to have adequate upper body strength to support your entire body. This may not be a problem for a young, fit person, but it may be a problem for an older, sedentary person. Six to eight training sessions geared to strengthening the upper body before surgery can make a real difference in helping to build up those muscles.

CHAPTER 7

Open-Knee Surgery

Both my knees were horribly arthritic. My life had become very restricted—I was in constant pain. Walking was an effort; dancing, which I used to love, was out of the question. I couldn't even shop anymore. I couldn't spend the day walking around the mall. I found myself sitting down a lot. I'm only fifty-five, but I was feeling like I was an old lady. I was scared about having knee replacements, but the prospect of spending the rest of my life like this was even scarier.

Joan, who had double knee replacement surgery

In most cases, arthritis can be controlled by a good exercise rehabilitation program and the judicious use of nonsteroidal anti-inflammatory drugs and other over-the-counter and home remedies. If symptoms persist, an arthroscopic procedure known as a "washout" may help provide temporary relief by removing debris (loose pieces of articular cartilage) that can cause inflammation and discomfort. However, for some patients, conservative therapies don't work. Their arthritis may progress to the point where they are in great pain and their mobility is severely impaired. In these cases, two types of open-knee procedures may be considered: osteotomy, in which the joint is surgically realigned, and a total knee replacement, which involves the insertion of a prosthetic knee.

Unlike arthroscopy, which can be performed through a tiny incision in the skin, open-knee surgery involves making a large incision (between 6 and 8 inches) in the skin and deeper tissues of the knee; it is major surgery that requires a substantial recovery period. Although we have made spectacular advances in recent years—notably in total knee replacements—surgery is not to be undertaken lightly. You should be thoroughly informed about the risks and the benefits, which I will be outlining in this chapter. Very often, the decision to have surgery may be more of a personal one than a medical one. You must decide when you have had enough pain and discomfort and when your life has been so adversely affected by your knee problems that you are ready to undertake the rigors of an arduous operation.

Although knee surgery is rarely an emergency procedure, there are times when the need for surgery is more pressing than others, notably in the case of a severe knock-kneed deformity. If a patient has this deformity, we will often recommend surgery sooner as opposed to later. The reason is simple: the peroneal nerve runs down the outside of the leg. In the case of a very severe knock-kneed deformity, the nerves can become relaxed and may start to sag. If the deformity is corrected, however, and the joint is realigned, the nerves are suddenly stretched back to a normal position, which can cause nerve damage and can lead to a loss of foot function. (The peroneal nerve can accommodate some gradual stretching, but sudden stretching can lead to damage, and we don't know exactly how much stretching is tolerable.) Therefore, we try to do corrective surgery before the knock-kneed deformity becomes too severe. In the case of severe bowlegs, we can wait longer to correct the problem because the nerves are being gradually stretched along with the deformity, and thus restoration of normal alignment relaxes the nerve.

Osteotomy

Before total knee replacements, osteotomy was the only surgical treatment for severe arthritis. Today, it is not performed as often as it used to be, yet it is still a relatively common surgery. (For every fifty to seventy-five total knee replacements that are performed, there is one osteotomy.) As the articular cartilage that lines the joint becomes worn down, it can destroy the normal alignment of the joint, resulting in knock-knees or bowlegs. Putting weight on the damaged area can be painful, which can severely hamper mobility. In an osteotomy, the surgeon cuts away bone from either the tibia or the femur to realign the leg, thus shifting the weight off the damaged area and onto an area of cartilage that is still intact. However, osteotomy is only successful for minimal deformities of not more than 10 degrees valgus (bowleg) or varus (knock-kneed). If the deformity is more serious, it will require a total knee replacement.

An osteotomy is performed under general anesthesia. Very often, plates, screws, or staples are required to set the bone, and they may have to be removed 18 months later. Osteotomy is performed as an inpatient procedure and patients can expect to spend up to three days at the hospital. Recovery from an osteotomy is not easy: it often requires wearing a cast for 6 weeks or more, depending on fixation, and it may take up to a year to resume normal activities. An exercise rehabilitation program is an important part of the healing process.

The success rate for osteotomy (which we define as pain-free mobility) is reasonably good: in the first 2 years, about 90 percent of all patients will report a marked improvement. However, that number quickly falls off to 75 percent at 5 years and 50 percent at 10 years. Some osteotomies have a better prognosis than others. Usually, in the case of a bowlegged deformity, osteotomy is done on the tibia or shinbone. In the case of a knock-kneed deformity, the osteotomy is done on the femur or thigh bone. Femoral osteotomies are more difficult for the surgeon to perform and are not as successful as tibial osteotomies. There is a relatively high rate of complications with osteotomy: between 2 and 8 percent of all patients will develop some kind of problem, which can include infection, nerve damage, and blood vessel damage.

Theoretically, the good news is, once you are thoroughly healed, you can resume normal activities. Unlike total knee replacement, there are no restrictions as to what you can do. The bad news is, for about half of all patients, osteotomy is a temporary procedure; after 10 years, they will require a total knee replacement.

Total Knee Replacement

The four goals of total knee replacement are freedom from pain, stability, adequate range of motion for the activities of daily living, and a durable prosthesis, that is, a new knee joint that will work for years to come. For the overwhelming majority of patients (approximately 90 to 95 percent), those goals are achievable.

In 1992, the latest figures available, there were 167,000 total knee replacement procedures performed in the United States. Total knee replacement has become the gold standard for the treatment of severe arthritis. Its success is nothing short of spectacular: 95 percent of all patients enjoy pain-free walking for at least 15 years after surgery. The database is growing every year and it might be closer to 20 years by 1996. The prosthesis, which has been refined and perfected over the past two decades, has proven to be strong and stable, so strong that many knee replacement patients are not just walking, they are dancing, playing golf, playing doubles tennis, and although we usually don't encourage it, some are even skiing (cross-country and downhill). As good as a prosthesis may be, it is not a real knee and cannot withstand the same forces as a real knee. Patients with knee replacements are instructed not to partake in competitive sports such as basketball or football, which put enormous stress on the knee, and we don't recommend running or singles tennis. Considering that many patients who have had this procedure couldn't walk without a crutch or a walker before the surgery, these restrictions are relatively minor. It must be stressed, however, that we still don't know exactly how aggressive the total knee athlete can be, but new studies suggest that they can probably engage in more vigorous activity than previously believed. The data are constantly being reassessed: one preliminary study suggests that we are being too conservative with the activity levels of our total knee patients.

Total knee replacement is performed under epidural anesthesia, in which anesthesia is injected into the lower back. (With an epidural, painkiller is injected in the spinal canal, but unlike spinal medication, the medicine does not go into the spinal fluid; rather, it bathes the nerves that run down the legs. There is less risk of residual headache as there is with a spinal, and the patient is much less groggy when the medication wears off.) This is preferable to general anesthesia because there is less blood loss. The leg is also wrapped in a tourniquet to control bleeding. In addition, the patient is given supplemental Valium or similar medication to induce sleep. During the operation, the leg muscles are completely relaxed, which makes it easier for the surgeon to move the leg around.

The operation for the total knee replacement takes between 1 and 2 hours, not including waiting time, induction of anesthesia, setting up, and prepping the knee. Complicated cases may take even longer. During the procedure, the surgeon must cut away the diseased bone, removing about 2 to 3 centimeters of bone from the joint, and must balance the ligaments in position to accommodate the prosthesis. The replacement knee consists of three components: a metal femur made from chrome cobalt or titanium, a patella made from a high-density polyethylene, and either a plastic tibia or a half-plastic, half-metal tibia. Usually, a young, active patient will receive the more expensive plastic–metal combination because it is stronger and able to withstand greater force.

The knee replacement must be contoured to fit the individual bones and put in position for alignment. During surgery, the surgeon must constantly flex and extend the knee, putting it through a full range of motion to make sure that the replacement knee works as well as a real knee. First, the surgeon uses trial components to get the correct fit, and then the real knee replacement is cut to the precise specifications and cemented into place. After knee replacement surgery, patients are hospitalized for 4 to 7 days or until they can bend their knee to 90 degrees. Rehabilitation is critical for a full recovery, which can take anywhere from 6 months to a year, depending on the age and condition of the patient and his commitment to exercise.

Possible Complications

As good as total knee replacement is, it is not without risk. Possible complications include infection (in less than 1 percent of all cases), nerve damage (which is more likely to affect a bad valgus knee deformity), dislocation, subluxation, fracture and loosening of the patella component (less than 2 percent), and, more rarely, the dislocation of the tibial or femoral component. Severe problems such as phlebitis (blood clots), heart attack, and stroke are also possible but extremely rare. A small number of patients may experience pain after surgery for no apparent reason. Skin numbness is another problem that can occur, and although it may be annoying to the patient, it is not a major complication. As a rule, I insist that patients who undertake this procedure be in good health, and in fact, patients are required to be examined by an internist within 2 weeks prior to surgery. Although there is a risk of aggravating cardiovascular problems during surgery, there is also ample evidence that living in chronic pain can put a major stress on the heart. Therefore, some doctors may approve a heart patient for a knee replacement if they feel that the benefits derived from the finite risks of surgery outweigh the risks of living in continuous pain. Heart patients may be monitored at an intensive care unit or a critical care unit overnight following surgery.

Although the component parts of the knee replacement are constantly being improved, over time, they may wear out or loosen. In some cases, they may fracture due to a traumatic injury, such as a car accident. In 1992, some 13,000 revision surgeries were performed. Revision surgeries are not as successful as first surgeries: studies show that about 80 to 85 percent of all patients will have pain-free mobility up to 15 years following second surgeries. (Patients who have total knee replacement surgery after osteotomies also have an 80 to 85 percent success rate.)

Given the success of the total knee replacement, why are osteotomies performed at all? This is a good question and one that is being debated in the medical community. The conventional wisdom is, osteotomy may be preferable for younger patients because it retains their own bone and joint and does not require the insertion of a prosthesis that might wear out. In addition, once the patient is healed, she can do whatever she likes, including competitive sports. The cost of both procedures is roughly the same in terms of the surgeon's fees and hospital bills; however, in the total knee surgery, there is the added cost of the prosthesis, which is about $2,000 to $3,500. However, given the fact that osteotomy is temporary and harder on the patient, many physicians are rethinking their position on the validity of osteotomies. If present trends continue and the total knee replacements become even better and longer lasting, there will be a natural evolution in favor of total knee procedures.

After Surgery

"I was in a lot of pain after surgery, but you know what? I was in a lot of pain before surgery!"

After surgery, you will wake up in the recovery room feeling groggy and will probably be in pain as the epidural wears off. However, you should be given adequate medication to control the pain. Many hospitals—mine included—use patient-controlled analgesia, which allows the patient to self-medicate as needed. (There is a safety mechanism to prevent overmedication.) Throughout your hospital stay, you will be given painkillers and an ice pack to help ease the pain. Given the extent of the surgery, it might seem as if the patients would be writhing in pain, but the fact is, most are not. Most are well able to tolerate it, and I think the reason is that people who have had severe arthritis have learned to live with pain. Now at least they have some hope that their pain will end.

Your knee will be covered in a large dressing with a drain for normal postoperative bleeding. Immediately following surgery, you will be started on Coumadin or some other anticoagulant, depending on your physician's preference, to prevent blood clots. When you are fully alert, you will be moved to your room to begin your recovery. Your leg will be swollen from the thigh down to the ankle. Within 3 to 4 days after a knee replacement, many patients will develop big black and blue marks on their buttocks and calf. This is normal and usually resolves itself within a few weeks. The sutures used to close the leg are removed in about 3 weeks following surgery. Over the next 6 months, your knee will swell up periodically.

Although the knee looks pretty awful after surgery, rest assured that within a year or two, all that will be left to remind you of your operation is a very thin white line that is barely noticeable.

After being released from the hospital, most patients will require some kind of home care assistance (on average 4 to 6 hours daily for at least 3 days a week) for the first 4 weeks or so. An older or disabled patient may require more help. Many patients are able to drive in about 6 to 8 weeks, and most are back at work within 6 weeks but may be walking with a cane. Some may return to work as early as 2 weeks, and some may require additional time off.

Caution Almost all patients will have a low-grade temperature (100 to 101 degrees) for 7 to 10 days (sometimes longer), a mildly swollen knee for anywhere from 6 weeks to 6 months, and increased skin warmth for up to 12 months. Wound drainage after 5 to 7 days is worrisome as is unusually prolonged pain, which should be evaluated by an experienced surgeon. He must ascertain whether it is a reflection of something gone wrong or whether it is related to your pain threshold.

Rehabilitation Training for Total Knee Replacement Surgery

Rehabilitation programs vary somewhat from patient to patient and from hospital to hospital. However, this section will give you some idea of what to expect from a typical rehabilitation program for total knee replacement. In general, the rehabilitation plan for a total knee replacement takes an average of 6 to 12 months before you are fully recovered, which means being able to function pain-free. Our program at the Insall Scott Kelly Institute is divided into three phases.

Phase 1

The first 6 weeks following surgery is the acute phase of rehabilitation. The initial goal is to help you go from a horizontal position to a vertical, upright position, ideally walking with only a cane. We also try to help you return to a good range of knee motion.

Within the first 6 months after surgery, the knee is often swollen, which can inhibit motion. Getting the knee joint moving is our first priority. As soon as possible following surgery—sometimes even in the recovery room—our patients are put on a continuous passive motion (CPM) machine, which constantly bends their knees in an elevated position as they lay in bed. The use of a CPM machine is somewhat controversial in that some studies have shown that there is very little difference in the outcomes of patients who use this machine and those who don't. In our experience, however, the use of the CPM machine is beneficial for several reasons, and we recommend that patients use it for several weeks after surgery. (In fact, we arrange for them to rent one for their homes.) First, some studies show that the CPM machine may help prevent blood clots. Second, patients are most disturbed by a stiff, immobile leg, which can hurt at the slightest movement. The CPM machine appears to help prevent the leg from stiffening, which in turn helps the patient develop a better range of motion early on. Some of the positive effect of the CPM machine may be psychological: if the patient sees that she can move her knee with the help of the machine, she may feel more inclined to try to do it herself.

Many patients tend to flex the operated knee for comfort. If kept in a flexed position continuously, it can hamper healing. Therefore, to prevent a flexed contraction, we instruct our patients to place the foot and ankle of their operated leg onto a towel roll or a towel pancake, elevating their lower limb. This position promotes knee extension, which, in turn, speeds up the healing process.

During the first week, you may also be put on an electrical stimulation machine, which makes the muscles contract and, thus, pumps fluid out of the knee. In addition, a physical therapist helps you to bend the knee on your own, and you may do other simple exercises. (See page 171 for specific exercises for rehabilitation for total knee replacement surgery.)

By the end of the first week, our goal is to have you bending your knee to about 80 to 90 degrees. If you can achieve this degree of flexibility, you should be able to walk out of the hospital on your own with the aid of a cane or a walker. In addition, you should be able to perform such basic tasks as getting in and out of the bathtub. If you have special needs, for example, if you must be able to walk up a flight of stairs at home, be sure to tell your physical therapist. You will need to practice walking stairs before you can return home.

Once you are discharged from the hospital, you will need some kind of help at home for the first few weeks. Mild pain analgesics may be required, but the need for medication should be reduced as time passes. Usually, by the sixth week, the pain begins to diminish, and you are able to do more things independently. During this period, you will continue on the CPM machine at home and will do mild strengthening exercises, such as straight leg raises and using a stationary bicycle. If you can, you will begin rehabilitation as an outpatient at the hospital or center in your neighborhood. Physical therapy is essential to return to normal strength and range of motion. You must commit to 3 days a week for at least 45 minutes a session. (If you are ill or severely disabled, a physical therapist may be sent to your home.)

Phase 2

Between 6 weeks and 6 months, the emphasis of rehabilitation shifts from simple exercises that can be done sitting or lying down to functional exercises that help return you to a functional lifestyle. *Functional* is the operative word. For example, an active patient who wants to return to cross-country skiing will have different exercises and goals than an older, arthritic patient whose primary goal is to be able to run her household. While the active patient is working out on a ski machine, the older arthritic one may be given instruction on how to do common household tasks, such as making a bed in a joint-sparing way or how to safely climb on a step stool to reach for something in a cabinet. By 6 months, you should be able to function fairly normally and hopefully are back to the way you used to be—or even better—than you were before your disability. It's not unusual for patients to say that after 6 months of rehabilitative therapy, they are in better physical shape than they have ever been. The challenge is maintaining that level of physical fitness.

Phase 3

After 6 months, during the final phase of rehabilitation, you should be motivated enough to do the necessary exercises on your own at home or at a gym. However, and I can't stress this enough, rehabilitation never really ends. Any patient who undergoes major knee surgery must understand that for the best result, he must make a lifetime commitment to exercise.

Caring for Your New Knee

Your knee prosthesis is designed for the activities of daily living, not for the rigors of vigorous sports. Usually patients are allowed to walk as much as they want, to play golf and doubles tennis. Activities that promote the risk of fracture or other injuries should be avoided. To be on the safe side, check with your physician before embarking on any activities. Before dental work or surgery, let your doctor or dentist know that you have knee replacement: you will need to take antibiotics to prevent infection before undergoing any "dirty" procedure that can introduce bacteria into the bloodstream. (We really don't know how long patients must take prophylactic antiobiotics. There are several on-going studies assessing this situation, and our recommendations might change after the data are complete.)

Keep in mind that your new knee contains pieces of metal

that might set off the metal detector at airport security points. Remember to alert the security personnel, or you may have difficulty boarding a plane.

Immediately after working out, apply ice wrapped in a plastic bag and a small towel to your knee to prevent swelling. Elevate your leg when you are sitting. Elevate your leg on two pillows (under your ankle) when you are asleep. Never place anything under your knee in the acute phase of rehabilitation. After your motion phase is completed, with your doctor's permission, you may place a pillow under your knee for comfort.

CHAPTER 8

All About Kids' Knees

Children are not merely miniature adults. As their bodies grow and develop, they have unique problems that often are misunderstood or overlooked even by the most concerned parents. This chapter will help parents to understand their children's knee problems better and distinguish normal growth and development from signs of trouble.

Early Childhood: When Normal Looks Wrong

From infancy to adulthood, as the body grows and develops, the knees go through many changes. Very often, during these formative years, what looks abnormal is actually normal. Consequently, many parents become unduly alarmed about variations in their children's alignment. The good news is, we've learned in recent years that for growing youngsters, there is a wide range of "normal," and what we used to think of as major "problems" are, more often than not, insignificant.

One of the most confusing issues for parents is their children's knee alignment. In adults, the normal alignment of the knee is a slight inward angulation (valgus). Infants, however, are born with a bowlegged deformity called *genu varum*, and by eighteen months, most children are in-toeing. By the time a child is between the ages of two and four, the legs angle in the opposite direction, resulting in knock-knees (valgus). As children continue to develop, the knock-knees may become less pronounced.

In the past, alignment problems such as knock-knees and in-toeing were taken very seriously. Many children were put in splints at night—the infamous Dennis Browne bars—and forced to wear ugly corrective shoes. Some were forced to perform hours of exercise each day to correct the deformity. Not only were these treatments ineffective (studies showed that none of them altered growth patterns), but we now know that in 95 percent of all cases, knock-knees correct themselves. This is not to say that parents should ignore the problem. A child with knock-knees should be evaluated every 6 months by his physician just to be sure that he is developing normally. In some cases, what appears to be a knee problem could actually be a congenital hip abnormality. In rare cases, the problem could be a growth disorder, such as Blount's disease, in which one side of the growth center of the bone grows but the other doesn't, resulting in a severe bowleg deformity. Blount's disease primarily affects children between the ages of one and three, and an adolescent form affects children older than eight. This condition is more common in the Caribbean than in the United States, and often requires the surgical realignment of the bones.

Although parents should be aware of their child's alignment irregularity, they should not focus on it, nor should they worry their child about it. There's one thing that parents can do that may help: they can try to encourage their child to refrain from sleeping with their feet under them—kids love to sleep in a curled-up position, and this may exacerbate the knock-knees. However, I want to stress that there's no reason to drive your child crazy about this; simply make the suggestion and let your child do this on his own.

In-toeing is another variation on alignment that greatly disturbs parents but shouldn't. There's no evidence that in-toeing is harmful; in fact, some of the best athletes in the world intoe. Just start watching track stars and basketball and football players, and you'll be amazed by the amount of in-toeing. There's some evidence that it may actually help you run faster!

There are times, however, when a child should be checked by a knowledgeable physician. If a child suddenly becomes bowlegged at age five or if there is a major change in alignment that appears to be abnormal, consult your pediatrician. Although it is rare in the developed world, rickets, a disease due to nutritional deficiency, could also result in abnormal bone growth. In extremely rare cases, a bone growth problem could be due to a tumor or infection.

Parents should be especially wary of a diagnosis of a fractured patella. The patella has two and sometimes three growth centers. In a small percentage of the population (2 to 5 percent), one of the growth centers might not fuse to the patella, which on X ray will look like a fracture, but it's actually normal. It's often overdiagnosed as a fracture in children, but keep in mind that a fractured patella is extremely rare in children. Very likely, it is a misdiagnosis.

Middle Childhood

As kids grow up and become more active, they're more prone to injury. Falls on the playground and cut knees are commonplace occurrences. In most cases, an injured knee will stop bleeding within 10 to 15 minutes and will not require any treatment other than cleaning the wound. Putting pressure on the injury is usually enough to stop the bleeding. However, if the bleeding persists or if the cut appears to be so deep that it may require stitches, see your pediatrician immediately. Although a scraped knee can be painful, rest assured that the cut is not in a location where a child could hurt a major vessel.

Even if the bleeding persists, it is probably due to a superficial vein or artery.

If your child falls on her knee and is in a great deal of pain, you can try to get her to stand up and see if she can walk. Don't worry about inflicting further damage, whatever damage there is has already occurred. If it is a serious injury, the leg will probably go into spasm, thus preventing further movement. Let your child try to move her leg through a normal range of motion, gently flexing and extending it without putting weight on it. If she can move it without pain, encourage her to walk. In general the ability to have a full range of motion and bear weight is an indication that it is only a minor injury. However, if there was a loud pop when the injury occurred (signifying a ligament or meniscal injury) or swelling develops within 15 to 20 minutes after the injury, take your child to an orthopedist for further evaluation.

If your child complains of knee pain and to your knowledge has not sustained an injury, have her looked at by an orthopedist. The problem may not be a knee problem at all—very often hip pain can be referred to the knee. Sometimes a child may have a problem and not articulate it. Children younger than seven may be unable to localize their pain. If you notice something amiss, for example, if your child is suddenly limping or refuses to walk, have her examined by a doctor. Even if your child says she's okay, there's a reason why she's limping. It may be a simple sprain, or it could be a back problem or a foot injury, but whatever it is, you should know about it.

Growth Plate Fractures

Most injuries involving children are due to minor trauma, usually involving soft tissue, such as muscle pulls or strained ligaments. Over time, these injuries generally heal on their own. In rare instances, a heavy force to a bone may result in a fracture or break. Generally, the treatment for fractures is no different for children than adults. Depending on the type of break, the leg is either put in a cast (closed reduction) or the bone is surgically reset (open reduction internal fixation), which can include the use of screws and plates.

However, there is one major difference between breaks in children and adults: children are still growing. In fact, the skeleton usually grows until the age of fourteen for girls and seventeen for boys. New bone is produced on growth plates that are located on specific sites on every bone. The growth plate (epiphyseal plate) connects the epiphysis (part of the bone closest to the joint) to the metaphyses. The growth plate is thus a transition from normal bone to the metaphyses, which eventually becomes the shaft of the bone. If an injury occurs on a growth plate on one leg, that leg could stop growing while the other continues to grow, resulting in legs of uneven length. In some cases, an injury to a growth plate could result in uneven growth on the same leg: one part of the leg grows normally, but the other doesn't, which causes the leg to grow in a curve instead of a straight line.

The symptoms of a growth plate fracture (also called *Salter fractures*) are pain and tenderness. A growth plate fracture is diagnosed with a stress X ray, a regular X ray that is performed while the technician or physician stresses the injured area as if he was performing a ligament stress test. If there is a growth plate fracture, the growth plate will open up upon stress, which will be detected on the X ray.

If the fracture is serious, open reduction internal fixation is required to put the bone back into normal position, although this is not without risk. Putting plates and screws across a growth plate can cause further damage, but it is a necessary risk if the fracture is to be repaired.

Osteochondritis Dessicans

Osteochondritis dessicans (OCD) and juvenile osteochondritis dessicans (JOCD) are separate problems that develop from stress fractures of the subchondral bone. JOCD, which develops as a result of an interruption of the blood supply to the subchondral bone, will heal in about 50 percent of cases. In this situation, the child's knee usually will not develop arthritic changes in adult life. In the remaining cases of JOCD that do not heal on their own, surgery will be required to put the piece back in position. Whether this can be accomplished arthroscopically or will require an arthrotomy is dependent on the fragment size. While the goal of treatment is to restore the joint surface to its original condition, often this cannot be accomplished. Diagnosis is most often made on standard X ray views but might well require an MRI or more sophisticated bone scan to delineate the size of the OCD lesion and its ability to heal. In addition to trying to pin the fragment back into position, in difficult cases the surgeon might consider a comparable bone cartilage fragment from a cadaver (allograft). There has also been some recent interest in cartilage cell implantation for large OCD defects, although more research is required to determine whether or not this is an effective treatment.

Playing It Safe

During middle childhood, children discover many different sports. Most kids can do whatever they want with few problems; however, there are some steps they can take to minimize their risk of knee injury. The following list reviews sports that are popular among children and the ways to play it safe.

In-line Skates

In-line skates are fun, and even better, the gliding motion diminishes the impact stress on the knee joints. However, falls are commonplace. To prevent serious injuries, make sure your child knows how to brake the skate before turning him loose on his own. All in-line skaters should wear a helmet and protective padding (on knees, legs, elbows, and hands). In-line skating is best done on a smooth surface far away from traffic.

Basketball

The most common problem with basketball is discomfort caused by overuse, so-called jumper's knee. The solution is simple: treat the pain with ice, and your child should not play for a few days until she feels better. The sudden movements involved in running and jumping can also cause ligament tears and meniscal injuries.

Bicycle Riding

Bicycle riding is kind to the joints and a great sport for kids as long as they remember to wear their helmets and knee pads.

Baseball

As with any other activity that involves running, jumping, and twisting, baseball can cause ligament or cartilage injuries. Kids are the most vulnerable to injury when they are sliding into a base. Rigid, immobile bases are especially problematic for the same reason it is dangerous to slide into a wall. The tremendous impact is often associated with a twisting movement that can result in a meniscal or ligament injury. Make sure your child knows how to slide correctly: he should avoid hitting the base with a sudden impact; rather, he should literally slide right into it, and the base should slide along with him.

Tennis

The major problem with tennis is pain due to overuse; kids who are pushed to practice several hours a day are especially vulnerable. Parents and coaches should keep in mind that professional athletes don't practice more than an hour or so daily, and neither should children. If a child complains of pain or discomfort, she should cut back on her practice time.

Soccer

Soccer is fine as long as it is played on a level field. The most common soccer injuries are muscle pulls due to dips in the playing surface.

Downhill Skiing

Skiing is a sport that is associated with significant injuries, especially to the ligaments and cartilage. Strong leg muscles can help guard against injury. Any child who wants to ski must have strong leg muscles before embarking on this sport.

Problems of the Adolescent and Teenage Athlete

More adolescents and teenagers than ever before are involved in some form of competitive sports. (Fifty percent of all boys and 25 percent of all girls ages eight to sixteen compete in an organized sports program sometime during the year.) Kids gain a great deal from participating in competitive sports: it's not only fun and good for self-esteem, but it can help them develop a lifetime habit of physical fitness. However, parents should be aware of the fact that can be a downside to competitive sports. Many kids are being pushed too far by coaches, parents, and perhaps even by themselves. As a result, we are seeing an increase in overuse injuries, which are caused by the chronic, repetitive stress related to sports, which can damage tissue, causing pain and discomfort. In athletic children, the knee is the most common site of overuse injury.

Many young athletes come to my office in great pain due to an overused and abused knee joint. In most cases, my prescription is the same: I tell the child and his parents that the problem can easily be solved by changing the child's approach to exercise. All too often, young athletes are not properly conditioned to participate in their sport. They don't pay enough attention to muscle strengthening and spend much too much time on aerobic exercise, such as jogging or running up and down steps (a real knee killer!) or practicing their sport for hours on end. It always amazes me that many young tennis players are expected to practice up to 6 hours a day, whereas adult professionals usually practice their game for only an hour a day. The pros know that excessive practice will not improve their game, but it will wear out their joints.

Usually, an overuse problem will disappear after the young athlete adapts a more balanced training program that strengthens the muscles without stressing the knee joint. It's also important for both coaches and parents to understand that even the most talented young athlete does not have the strength or endurance of an adult. Unlike adults, kids have underdeveloped bodies, and much of their energy is expended on growing. It is impossible for a growing child to amass the muscle strength of an adult. Therefore, a good coach must be aware of the limits of young athletes and should tailor their activities accordingly.

It is especially important for athletic activities to be properly geared to growing girls. Due to alignment differences, in many girls, the kneecap may sit off to the side. This doesn't mean that girls should avoid sports, but it does mean that athletic girls should avoid activities that constantly stress their knee joints. A girl can certainly run if she's on the track team; however, she should use other forms of exercise for conditioning that are kinder to her joints, such as biking, swimming, or weight lifting.

Osgood–Schlatter disease is the most common overuse injury of the knee of adolescent athletes. The condition is due to continual stress on the spot where the patellar tendon inserts into the tibial tubercle. Osgood–Schlatter disease is characterized by pain and/or tenderness at the patellar tendon and a prominent bump. In young children, there may be tenderness without a bump.

In the past, kids with Osgood–Schlatter disease were casted for about 6 months, which severely limited their activities. However, casting created new problems, so it's no longer a viable treatment. Today, the treatment for Osgood–Schlatter disease is simple: if the child is in pain, let her use ice to reduce the swelling and discomfort. Strengthening the muscles around the knee may also help relieve some of the stress on the patellar tendon. If your child can play her sport without being in too much discomfort, it's fine to let her play; she will not damage her knee.

If an adolescent or teenager is in continuous pain for whatever reason, a change in conditioning will often do the trick. However, if the young athlete continues to complain about pain, and his doctor can't find anything wrong, I think it's wise for the child to cut back on his sport for a while. It's important for parents to communicate the message that sports should be fun. If the child is in so much pain that playing his sport is not fun, I think it's time for the parents and the child to sit down and figure out what's really happening. Perhaps the child is pushing himself too much, or perhaps the parents are hoping that their son's athletic ability will garner a scholarship to college, and perhaps the child is feeling a great deal of pressure. Whatever it may be, if the child becomes preoccupied with pain, it's important for him to stop playing until he can enjoy the sport again.

In my opinion, it is never appropriate for children to take any kind of anti-inflammatory medicines or painkillers to play their sport. Kids should be told that all athletes will experience some degree of discomfort after a hard workout, and it's perfectly fine to use ice to relieve minor aches and pains. But if a child is in a great deal of pain, she should feel free to say to her parents or her coach, "My knee hurts too much today, I'm not going to play." If parents or coaches find that they are pushing medication on a child so that she can play, it's a sign that the child is being pushed in an unhealthy way.

CHAPTER 9

How Women's Knees
Are Different

Due to differences in anatomy, girls and women are at particular risk of sustaining knee injuries. Younger, active women appear to be more prone to sports injuries such as ligament tears. Older, sedentary women are more likely to sustain fractures on their legs or knees and are also more prone to develop severe arthritis. In fact, of the 167,000 total knee replacement surgeries performed in 1992, more than two-thirds were done on women. This chapter will explain why women are vulnerable and, most importantly, what women need to do to reduce their risk.

The Active Woman

When the modern Olympic Games were first organized at the turn of the century, women were excluded from participating in sports because it was believed to be "against the laws of nature." Times have changed for the better. Today, it seems perfectly natural to see women on the tennis courts, running marathons, working up a sweat in step classes, and even pumping iron at the local gym. This changing tide is especially dramatic among school-age girls. Since the adoption of Title

IX to the Education Amendments in 1972, all schools that receive federal funds are required to give girls equal access to sports or be denied funding. Since that law was passed, there has been an impressive 600 percent increase in female participation in high school sports. Although the growing numbers of girls and women involved in physical fitness is a positive change, all too often, they are embarking on strenuous activities without the proper preparation or understanding of their anatomy.

Due to their different reproductive roles, men and women have basic anatomical differences. These differences not only affect their reproductive systems, but have a profound impact on alignment, which ultimately affects the extensor mechanism, the group of muscles, tendons, and bones that are involved in bending the knee forward.

Alignment is the way your bones—from your hips down to your ankles—stack up in relation to each other. Bones must be aligned in such a way that allows for both stability and flexibility. A minor variation in alignment is not serious; however, if the alignment is truly out of whack, it could cause pain and discomfort. Most men have what we call 0 alignment, which means that the bones—from the hip bone to the femur to the patella to the tibia—are straight in relation to the midline of the body. Women, however, have a wider pelvis than men, which changes the alignment of both the bones and muscles. To accommodate the wider pelvis, a woman's femur turns slightly in toward the midline of the body, and her tibia turns slightly outward, making her slightly knock-kneed. To complicate the situation, the quadriceps—the four muscles on the front of the thigh that run down from the hip—angle out, which pulls the kneecap, or patella, slightly off to the side. As a woman moves her leg, the patella moves up and down and rotates in order to locate itself on the trochlea. If the patella is pulled too far off to the side, it can be pulled off its normal alignment, which can cause pain and discomfort. If the patella moves slightly off its grove, it's called a *subluxation;* if it's completely off its groove, it's called a *dislocation*. In severe cases, surgery may be necessary to get the patella back on track.

In women, patellar pain may be caused by this variation in alignment and may be not significant. An active woman who participates in sports or does other forms of exercise may find that her knees may at times feel achy or painful. It's often hard for patients to understand, but pain does not necessarily coincide with destruction. Sometimes, you just hurt. Nonmedical treatments, such as ice and the occasional use of over-the-counter nonsteroidal anti-inflammatory drugs may be enough to reduce the pain. Obviously, avoiding any activities that exacerbate discomfort is also wise. Women also often complain about cracking and creaking in their knees. This is nothing to worry about; it is due to the noise the kneecap makes when it glides up and down its track. Noise without swelling or the inability to move the leg is not serious and should be ignored.

This is not to say that women don't have real patellar problems; many do. Knee dislocations are more common among women than men. In fact, women appear to be more prone to chondromalacia, or softening of the articular cartilage, the cushion behind the kneecap.

The evidence is now mounting that women are much more likely to sustain an anterior cruciate ligament injury than men, particularly in sports that involve jumping and pivoting, such as basketball and soccer. Some experts theorize that women have smaller, laxer ligaments, which make them more injury prone. The increased rate of injury in women is probably due to a narrower "notch" on the femur, the origin of the ACL, which makes the ligament at greater risk for rupture.

Too Much Stretching, Too Little Conditioning

When it comes to muscle strength, women are at a disadvantage. Women have about 40 to 75 percent of the upper extremity muscle strength of men and 60 to 80 percent of the lower extremity strength. Given the fact that women have naturally weaker muscles and laxer ligaments, it would make sense for women to concentrate more on building muscle and less on stretching. However, just the opposite occurs. Girls and women flock to "stretch" classes and avoid muscle building because they believe that strength training will lead to big muscles that are unfeminine and unattractive (it won't). Stretching is useful only to warm up muscles and loosen up the joints prior to engaging in your sport and to cool down when you're done. A few minutes of stretching goes a long way in helping to keep you flexible; too much stretching can overcompress the joints and actually promote discomfort and sometimes injury. On the other hand, strong muscles—especially strong quadriceps—can actually prevent injuries. Very simply, if the muscles work harder, they can take some of the stress off the kneecap as well protect the cartilage, ligaments, bones, and other components of the knee joint.

When I talk about strength training for women, I'm not talking about working out until the muscles bulge in an unnatural way. A moderate strength training program can help tighten and tone muscles without adding much bulk. A case in point are ballet dancers, who have very strong muscles but are hardly muscle-bound. Several studies have shown that strength training may also help to prevent osteoporosis, the thinning of bone that can lead to fractures. To maintain strength, every woman should work out 3 or 4 days a week, between 30 and 45 minutes each session. For more information on the right kinds of strengthening exercises, see page 171.

Women who embark on any sport should be especially vigilant about getting their muscles in shape prior to playing their sport. Tennis and skiing are a lot of fun, and they can provide a good aerobic workout, but they are for recreation: they are not conditioning programs. Vigorous sports can put a great deal of pressure on the knee joint, and it is critical that the leg muscles are strong enough to withstand the added force. This is true for both men and women, but it is especially true for women because of their alignment problems.

Although I believe that women can engage in almost any sport, I think that women need to be aware that any activity that continually bangs up their kneecaps is likely to cause problems. Two activities that have become extremely popular in recent years—step training and stair machines—may not be the most knee-wise of activities. I usually don't recommend step machines or step classes for women because they put tremendous stress on the knee joint. Remember, each time you run up or down stairs, with each step you are exerting between seven and eight times your body weight through your knee joint. Although it may give you a great cardiovascular workout, it is sheer hell on your knees. In fact, orthopedic surgeons often joke that step machines are an orthopedist's annuity: if you use them often enough, at high enough resistance, it is inevitable that you will be paying us a visit. However, I would much prefer not to get patients from situations that are so clearly avoidable. (For information on how to use a step machine safely, see page 199.)

Running and jogging are also likely to cause knee discomfort in women. Due to their irregular alignment, women are more prone to develop "runner's knee," a common problem caused by overuse. If you are a passionate jogger or runner, I recommend that you run for speed rather than endurance. Over time, the continuous force on your knees will in all likelihood cause pain, if not destruction.

Very active girls and women often develop menstrual irregularities such as a longer than average menstrual cycle or the absence of menstrual bleeding. Studies have linked menstrual irregularities to a tendency to develop stress fractures, small, microscopic breaks in the bone that can be quite painful. Although we don't know the precise reason for the increased risk in stress fractures, numerous studies have shown that female athletes have lower levels of certain estrogens than normal, and estrogen plays a role in bone building. Menstrual irregularity in athletes can also lead to skeletal demineralization, or premature osteoporosis. Any active woman who has irregular periods should consult with her physician.

During pregnancy, many women complain of knee pain. This is due to an increase in weight gain that is necessary to nourish the fetus but also increases the force across the joint. Although this may be uncomfortable, it does not cause long-lasting damage, and the pain usually disappears after delivery.

Osteoporosis

About 24 million Americans have osteoporosis, which literally means porous bones; four out of five are women. Osteoporosis causes 1.5 million bone fractures each year. The hips, wrists, and spine are most vulnerable, but any bone, including the bones in the leg and knee, can be prone to fracture.

The precise cause of osteoporosis is unknown, but the damage that it can inflict on women is all too familiar. By age eighteen, bones reach about 95 percent of their maximum density, and by age twenty-five, both men and women have reached their peak bone mass. After age thirty-five, the body builds less bone to replace the loss of old bone. However, after menopause, bone loss is accelerated in women. Although men also lose bone, they lose it much more slowly. In addition, they have bigger bones to begin with, and this, combined with stronger muscles, helps protect them against fractures. In women, bone loss increases from less than 1 percent per year after age thirty-five to as much as 4 percent per year during the 5 to 10 years after menopause. Many experts believe that the reduction in estrogen somehow interferes with the body's ability to absorb dietary calcium, which, in turn, causes the bones to thin out. The big bones become more brittle and prone to fractures and breaks. If the bone is weak enough, even a relatively minor stress, such as picking up a small package, can fracture a bone in the spine. Or, in some cases, a fall that would not have been of any consequence could result in a broken patella or femur.

Some forms of osteoporosis may be hereditary. Women who are fair with a small build of Caucasian or Asian ancestry appear to be at greater risk. In addition, a family history of bone fractures may also increase the odds of developing osteoporosis. Recently, researchers have isolated a gene that they feel may be responsible for this potentially crippling disease. People who have this gene have different vitamin D receptors on their cells; vitamin D is crucial for the absorption of calcium.

Environmental factors also come into play. Smoking and excessive alcohol use have been linked to this bone-thinning disease. Women with a history of menstrual disorders, early menopause, or eating disorders may be more prone to fractures due to osteoporosis. In addition, some medications, including steroids, and illnesses, such as thyroid disorders, can promote osteoporosis. Diet may also be an important factor: girls who get an adequate amount of calcium during their bone-building years may be able to grow enough bone reserve to protect themselves in their later years. Keeping active after menopause is very important for a variety of reasons, not the least being that it is good for your bones. There is some evidence that exercise may also protect against osteoporosis. Several studies have shown that weight-bearing exercise, such as walking, working out with weights, and regularly using a cross-country ski machine, may help build up bone mass. (Unfortunately, non-weight-bearing exercise, such as swimming, does not.) In addition, a woman with a well-conditioned body is more surefooted, has stronger muscles, and is less likely to sustain a fall. (For specific knee strengthening exercises for women with osteoporosis, turn to page 171.)

As of yet, there is no cure for osteoporosis—we haven't yet figured out how to trigger the growth of new bone—and there are few effective treatments. There are only two drugs approved by the Food and Drug Administration for the treatment of osteoporosis: estrogen replacement therapy and salmon calcitonin. Estrogen or hormone replacement therapy (HRT), which is prescribed to millions of menopausal women, has been shown to stop bone loss in the years following menopause but is much less effective for women over the age of seventy-five. Estrogen, however, may increase the risk of developing breast and uterine cancers and is not safe for many women. The drug calcitonin, which is a hormone produced by the thyroid gland in humans and other animals, has been shown to stop bone loss and relieve the pain of fractured bones. Calcitonin is delivered by injection, and a nasal spray version of the drug, which is used in Europe, is currently being tested in the United States.

Although it is still controversial, some researchers believe that high levels of dietary calcium past menopause (1,500 milligrams daily) combined with 400 IU of vitamin D may help prevent bone loss. Fifteen hundred milligrams is the amount of calcium in about five glasses of skim milk or five servings of plain, nonfat yogurt, which is a lot for many women to swallow. Although there are other foods that are rich in this mineral, few women can get enough calcium through diet alone. Therefore, many physicians recommend a daily calcium supplement.

Women and Knee Surgery

A recent study conducted by researchers at Brigham and Women's Hospital in Boston compared the severity of symptoms of male and female patients with arthritis who underwent knee or hip replacement and laminectomy, a procedure in which portions of the vertebrae are removed to relieve pressure on the spinal cord. In each case, the researchers found that the women were in far worse shape than the male patients before having the surgery and had a greater degree of disability. However, the women did not have a higher rate of complications from the orthopedic surgery, and interestingly, women who underwent knee replacement actually fared better than men who had this procedure. The authors of the study weren't sure why women waited so long to have the surgery but suggested that since women are often the primary caregivers in a family, they are reluctant to take time away from their household to take care of themselves.

Although major surgery such as a total knee replacement should not be rushed into, older women should keep in mind that the longer they wait, the greater the risk of developing another ailment that might make them ineligible for surgery at a later date. In addition, many women may be spending years suffering needlessly, whereas the surgery would not only relieve their pain, but vastly improve their lifestyle.

CHAPTER 10

Playing It Safe: Preventing Sports Injuries

In recent years, the emphasis in exercise has been on cardio-vascular health. Any form of exercise that got the heart pump-ing and the pulse racing was considered to be beneficial. As a result, millions of Americans routinely run, jog, go to aerobics classes, and pound away on stair machines. Even when they're not officially exercising, countless numbers of people eschew elevators in favor of stairs or run when they can walk, all in the name of fitness. But as any orthopedist will tell you, there's a downside to the fitness fixation. Although exercise is a won-derful way to maintain overall health and well-being, some of the same activities that are good for the heart are extremely hard on the joints, especially the knees. In fact, the over-whelming majority of sports injuries occur in the legs, with about one-third of them directly affecting the knee. This is not to say that exercise is dangerous to your knees or that you should refrain from engaging in activities that you love—not at all. However, if you want to keep on enjoying your sport without injury, it's essential to learn how to exercise in a joint-sparing way.

When it comes to maintaining healthy knees, I advise pa-tients to divide their lives into the following three compo-nents.

Activities of daily living. During the course of a normal day, the average person takes between 12,000 and 15,000 steps. Each step exerts a force of up to two to five times your body weight through your knees, depending on whether you're walking on soft carpet or hard concrete. Every time you run or walk up stairs, you are exerting a force of up to eight times your body weight through your knee joint. The odds are, if you do this often enough, you're eventually going to cause discomfort to, if not destruction of, your knees. Don't sacrifice one part of your body for another. Save your cardiovascular conditioning for when you're actually exercising. Bypass the steps for the elevator when you can. (But if you have to walk up stairs, don't worry about it, just don't go out of your way to find them!)

Conditioning or muscle strengthening. Many people mistakenly believe that their sport is their conditioning, that is, they can run, jog, or play tennis without first building up their muscles. This may be true for kids, but once you hit twenty, it's a recipe for disaster. After about age twenty, muscles begin to slowly atrophy or weaken, and by middle age, the rate of atrophy rapidly accelerates. At any age, sports require strong leg muscles to cushion the force exerted through the knee joint. If your muscles are weak, the joint will have to bear too great a load on its own, which can lead to injury. If you want to participate in sports, a good muscle-strengthening program is not optional, it's essential. A good conditioning program should be low-impact and non-weight-bearing—no running, jumping, or anything else that sends shock waves through the knee joints. Working out with weights or using a stationary bicycle or cross-country ski machine 3 days a week, up to 45 minutes at a time, are excellent ways to condition your muscles without overstressing your knees.

Recreation. Your sport—whether it's walking, skating, or swimming—is for your enjoyment and well-being. It's good for your body and your head, but—and I can't stress this enough—it is not a conditioning program. You must be in good condition to play. It's also important to realize that some sports are more stressful on the knees than others. Sports that are high torque, that is, sports that require a great deal of twisting or rotation, such as basketball, running, skiing, and football, are harder on the knees than other sports. These types of activities should not be undertaken by people who are not in peak condition.

Preparing to Play

All sports require a 5- to 10-minute warm-up period to prepare the muscles for increased activity. Gentle stretching exercises are a good way to gear up your muscles. However, many people make the mistake of overstretching, which can actually hurt their knee joints. Never push or pull on your leg with your hands while you are stretching; it can result in a joint compression syndrome that can be quite painful. Let your leg do the work by itself. Avoid squatting during warm-ups; this position can put a great deal of pressure on the joint and can result in cartilage tears, especially among older people. (For information on the correct way to do warm-ups, see page 170.)

Popping Pills

At any age, you may feel some aches and pains during or after you're playing. An occasional twinge or ache is normal; being in excruciating pain is not. Your sport should not hurt. If an activity is causing a great deal of pain or discomfort to your knee, cut back or stop doing it. It may be a sign of an overuse injury, and very often, it will heal on its own with ice and rest. I don't recommend using painkillers to play a sport; if an activity is causing you enough discomfort that you need to pop a few pills to play, you should reevaluate your conditioning program. Chances are, you're not conditioned enough, you're not doing the right exercises, or you're doing them incorrectly. Whatever it is, you should not be masking your symptoms with medication.

The Right Gear

I think the best footwear on the market today are sneakers or athletic shoes. They are better fitted (many come in a wide selection of sizes and widths) and more cushioned than normal shoes, which can reduce the impact of the load exerted through the knee. Any of the top-of-the-line brands are fine; just be sure that the shoes fit well and are comfortable. If you have a tendency to turn over your ankle, a high-top sneaker may be better than a low-cut one.

Some people feel more comfortable and secure wearing an athletic brace around their knee while they are playing their sport, but this may cause more problems than it's worth. Although a brace may feel good while you are playing, if it's too tight, it can cause pain and discomfort afterward. The same is true for Ace bandages, which should not be used around the knee at all. If you do use a brace, be sure that it's one that has a hole or padding around the kneecap to prevent patellar–femoral joint compression. In most cases, if you don't have any pain or swelling, it's probably fine to use a brace. However, to be on the safe side, if you feel you may need a brace, I recommend that you consult with your physician. Keep in mind that there is no evidence that a brace will prevent injuries, and it is no substitute for building up your own muscle strength.

Tips on Knee Safety

Depending on which you sport you choose, your knees may be vulnerable to different types of injuries. Even under the best of circumstances, injuries will occur to even the most seasoned athletes. However, there are some simple steps that you can take to reduce your risk of injury. The following is an analysis of the potential pitfalls of each sport and how to prevent them.

Racket Sports

Racket sports—primarily tennis and racquetball—are high-torque activities that require a great deal of pivoting and rotation. Common injuries for racket sports include sprained ligaments, torn cartilage, and patellar dislocations. Racket sports are extremely popular among weekend athletes, people who do nothing all week long and think that an hour or two of tennis on the weekend will fulfill their exercise quota. Unfortunately, out-of-condition people are most prone to injuries. Racket sports should only be played by the very fit who have a regular conditioning program. Some books suggest that people can prevent racket sport injuries by changing their gait pattern; in other words, if they move differently, they won't get injured. This is nonsense. Gait pattern is a highly individual, complicated phenomenon that is dependent on such factors as the rotation of the hip, leg, knee, and foot. Everyone moves a little differently, and there is no right way or wrong way. Movement should be natural and spontaneous—it is not something that you can control, especially in the heat of a game. There is only one way to reduce the risk of knee injuries, and that is to build up muscle strength in your legs.

Soccer

Soccer is another high-torque activity that can result in torn cartilage, meniscal injuries, and sprained ligaments. The constant pivoting and twisting at high speed required by those who play this sport can cause microscopic tears of the menisci that may eventually cause pain; however, more serious ligament damage is also possible. Building up your leg muscles is one way to protect against injury. Playing on a level field is another. Very often, soccer injuries are caused when a foot accidentally lands in a pothole. If you play on an uneven field, be sure to check out the field before the game to pinpoint any particularly troublesome spots.

Snow Skiing

Snow skiing is one of the most dangerous sports for your knees. According to a recent report that appeared in the *Berkeley Wellness Letter,* out of the 5 million people who ski each year in the United States, some 25,000 will sustain a serious knee sprain. The anterior cruciate ligament is particularly vulnerable to injury due to the high speed of the sport combined with the twisting motion that can occur in the leg when a ski goes out of control. Some sports medicine experts believe that the higher, stiffer ski boots that are designed to protect against ankle injuries and broken legs may promote knee injuries by forcing the lower leg forward in a jump or fall, thus stressing the knee. Theoretically, this seems to make sense. I also believe, however, that there are also other reasons why skiers are particularly vulnerable to knee injuries. Skiing is usually done at high altitudes, resulting in decreased oxygen consumption—even the hardiest of athletes will fatigue more easily. In addition, because it is performed at high speed, skiing requires tremendous muscle coordination. If the muscles are not in peak condition, the ligaments will be overtaxed, which could result in sprains.

Skiing is not a sport that should be undertaken without substantial preparation. If you are not in peak condition, you need to embark on a muscle-strengthening program at least 6 weeks before a ski trip. Special attention should be paid to building up the quadriceps and the hamstrings. In my practice, I have noticed that young adults, especially those right out of college, are particularly vulnerable to ski accidents. Very often, people who had been athletic throughout their school years find that once they begin a job, they are no longer able to work out as often. Weeks may go by before they get to the gym, and their muscles begin to atrophy. When they go on a ski trip in this weakened state, they may mistakenly believe that they can do what they used to do, only to end the weekend with a sprained ligament or some other injury.

Basketball

For a poorly conditioned person, basketball is risky business. The constant pivoting and twisting typical of this sport can easily lead to knee injuries. There is also an equal risk that you may be injured by another player. Middle-aged people who typically play an occasional game on the weekend may try to do such tricky maneuvers as blocking the shot of another player. The only problem is, they are often two steps behind where they should be and may collide with the other player. My advice: don't dunk or do anything that requires a great deal of speed unless you are a well-conditioned, experienced player. For your protection, play with younger players: kids are usually able to block a shot cleanly, and while they may humiliate you on the court, they're not going to send you to the emergency room. Ditto for volleyball.

Football

A beautiful weekend, a couple of guys who haven't played in years start throwing around a football. They run, jump, and try to cut at high speed, and then, one of them goes down with a thud. Like other high-torque sports, football (even touch football) is not to be undertaken by people who are out of shape. If you want to play, start on a muscle-strengthening program several weeks before the game. Similar to soccer, be especially careful about playing on an uneven field. Also keep in mind that tackle football is only for the very young or very well-paid professionals.

Running and Jogging

Running is a high-stress sport for your knees, and although jogging is somewhat less stressful, it can still cause injury. Keep in mind that with every step you run or jog, you are pounding hundreds of pounds through your knee joints. This can be particularly punishing for people who have knee alignment problems or a history of ligament injuries. Runners must be scrupulous about maintaining muscle strength. Anyone who runs should be working out several times a week to keep in good condition. If you love to run, as many runners do, I advise people to run for speed and recreation rather than for endurance. By all means do your half-hour run every day if it makes you feel good, but don't go overboard. You don't have to run twenty marathons a year, you can run one or two. And when a marathon is over, there is no need to maintain the same pace as when you were in training. A common sense approach to running can help to prevent injuries.

Swimming

For most people, swimming is a joint friendly sport that gives a good cardiovascular workout without beating up their knees. However, some people with congenitally malaligned kneecaps (kneecaps that go off to the side) may find that they have pain when they try to do the breast stroke or whip kicks. Listen to your body: the pain is telling you that this is too stressful for your knees, and you should find another sport.

Bicycling

Bicycling is safe as long as the bike is made to accommodate your body and not vice versa. Be sure to set the seat height so your knees are not hyperextended or bent more than 90 degrees. Competitive cyclists may lock their feet onto the pedals to improve speed. This position may cause additional stress on the knee joint, which can be painful. If you find that you are in pain, try changing the position of your feet to stress-relieve the joint.

Baseball

Baseball is a reasonably knee friendly sport with three caveats. First, rigid bases are dangerous: use soft, movable bases that "give" when you slide into them. A short, sudden stop could result in a ligament or meniscal injury. Gradually slide into the base. Second, catchers who are constantly squatting are prone to kneecap problems. An out-of-shape weekend player who spends hours squatting may be particularly vulnerable. Third, beware of an uneven playing field. A pothole or dip in the ground could result in injury.

Walking

Although walking is viewed as a benign exercise, it's important to remember that it can still stress the knees. People who walk for exercise should also condition their leg muscles. They also have to use their common sense. If they find that walking 4 miles a day results in knee pain, then perhaps they should cut back to 2 miles a day and make up the difference with a more joint-sparing exercise, such as a cross-country ski machine or a stationary bicycle.

APPENDIX

Exercise Rehabilitation Programs

General Strengthening Program
for Everyone

Throughout this book, I have spent a great deal of time describing common knee injuries and how they are treated. I don't want to leave you with the impression, however, that knee injuries are inevitable. They most certainly are not. As I stated earlier, one of the primary reasons that I am writing this book is to show how many common knee injuries can be prevented, and the best way to prevent knee injuries is to follow a good muscle-strengthening program. With the help of Robert Gotlin, the physician-in-charge of Beth Israel Hospital's North Division, Orthopaedic and Sports Spine Rehabilitation, we have devised a program specifically geared to help prevent knee problems. All of our recommended exercises are simple and can be done right at home or at any health club. Do these exercises at least three times a week for 45 minutes at a time. By following our program, you will not only keep your leg muscles strong and flexible, but you should be able to avoid many common knee problems.

Your exercise program should consist of the following three components:

Warming Up.   Before beginning your strengthening exercises, you must warm up your muscles in preparation for your workout. There are several excellent ways to warm up. We recommend using a stationary bicycle for 5 to 10 minutes (if you don't own a stationary bicycle, most health clubs have several to choose from), running in place for 5 minutes, or using a treadmill at the gym or health club for 5 to 10 minutes (short steps only) at a comfortable pace (see exercise 15).

Stretching.   Five or ten minutes of gentle stretching can help improve flexibility. We recommend the hamstring stretch (exercise 6) and the supine hamstring stretch (exercise 7).

Strengthening Exercises.   We have selected some basic exercises that are designed to maintain strong leg muscles and healthy knees (exercises 14a,b,c,d, 15, or 19a,b,c,d, 22, and all water exercises: 11, 12, 13). Some of these exercises (bicycling and stepping) can also can help to maintain good cardiovascular health, which is an essential part of any exercise program.

A word of caution: If you have any health problems or are over age forty, be sure to check with your physician before doing any of the exercises mentioned in this book. Most people can exercise safely with few problems; however, if you experience any of the following symptoms during your workout, discontinue the exercises and check with your physician:

- Light-headedness or dizziness.
- Nausea.
- Chest discomfort.
- Shortness of breath.
- Fatigue.
- Profuse sweating.

Rehabilitation Programs for
Special Problems

Meniscal Injuries, Injuries to the Articular Cartilage, and Arthritis. For these problems, we recommend the following exercises: 1, 2, 3, 4, 5, 6, 7, 8, 9, 10a, b, 11, 12, 13, 14a,b,c, 15a,b, 17, 18, 19a,b,c, 20, 22, 23.

Ligament Injuries and Reconstruction. For these problems, we recommend the following exercises: 1, 2, 3, 4, 5, 6, 7, 8, 9, 10a, b, 11, 12, 13, 14a,b,c, 15, 16, 17, 18, 19a,b,c,d, 20, 21a,b, 22, 23, 24, 25.

Patellar Injuries. For patellar injuries, we recommend the following exercises: 3, 4, 5, 6, 8, 9, 10, 11, 12, 13, 14a,b,c, 15a,b, 16, 17, 18, 19a,b,c,d, 20, 22, 23.

Total Knee Replacement. For total knee replacement, we recommend the following exercises divided into two phases. Phase I is up to the first 6 weeks postsurgery. Phase II is up to the first 6 months postsurgery.
Phase I: 1, 2, 3, 4, 5, 6, 7, 8, 10b, 15a, 17.
Phase II: 4, 5, 11, 12, 13, 15b, 17, 18, 19a,b,c,d.

Osteoporosis. We recommend the following exercises for people with osteoporosis: 11, 12, 13, 15, 16, 17, 20, 22, 23, 24.

Note: All exercises should be done with a gentle, fluid motion. Sudden twists and jolts can cause fragile bone to crack. Although the water exercises listed above are excellent for developing cardiovascular endurance, they are not weight-bearing exercises and will not help to maintain and build bone.

1   HEEL SLIDE

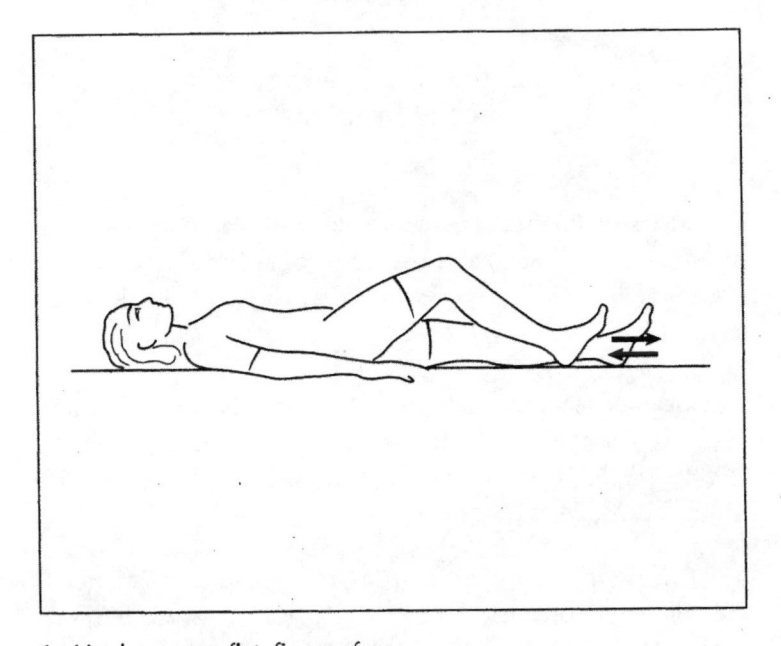

1. Lie down on a flat, firm surface.
2. Gently slide one leg toward your chest while keeping your heel on the floor. Bend your knee as much as you can, as long as there is no pain. If you are in pain, do not bend more than 90 degrees.
3. Straighten your leg by sliding your heel forward.
4. Repeat exercise 10 times. Do 2 more sets of 10.
5. Repeat exercise with other leg.

2 ASSISTED KNEE EXTENSION

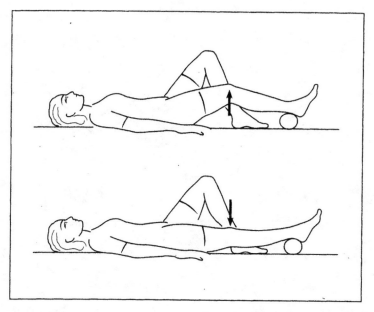

1. Lie down on a flat, firm surface. Keep one leg straight, bend the other.
2. Place a small bolster (a rolled-up towel) under the ankle of the straight leg.
3. Push down from the bottom of the thigh of the straight leg right above the knee. (You are contracting your quadriceps muscles.) The goal is to extend the knee just as much as it takes to straighten the leg. Be careful not to hyperextend.
4. Hold for a count of 6. Repeat 10 times. Do 2 more sets of 10.
5. Repeat exercise with other leg.

3 TERMINAL KNEE EXTENSION

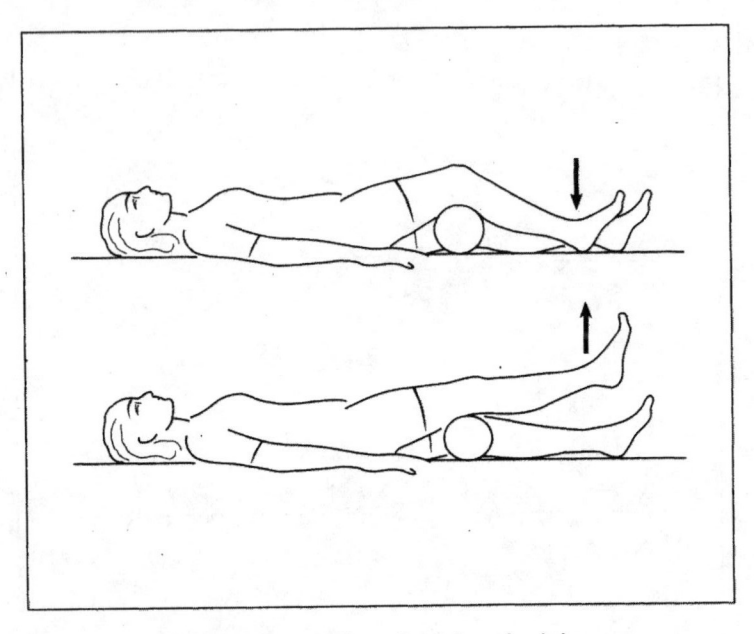

1. Lie down on a flat, firm surface. Straighten both legs.
2. Place a bolster (a rolled-up towel) under the hamstring muscle, which is just above the knee.
3. Straighten your knee to extend your leg. The goal is to extend your knee just as much as it takes to straighten the leg. Be careful not to hyperextend the knee.
4. Hold for 30 seconds. Repeat exercise 10 times. Do 2 more sets of 10.
5. Repeat exercise with other leg.

4 STRAIGHT LEG RAISE

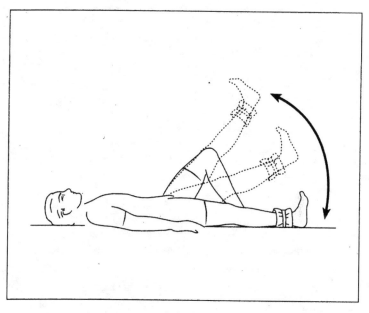

1. Lie down on a flat, firm surface. Bend one leg, straighten the other leg.
2. Slowly raise and lower the extended leg. Take 4 counts to raise the leg and 8 counts to lower the leg. (Or in other words, it should take twice as long to lower the leg as it does to raise it.)
3. Repeat exercise 10 times. Do 2 more sets of 10.
4. As you get stronger, you can add 3- to 5-pound ankle weights to make the exercise more challenging.
5. Repeat exercise with other leg.

SPECIAL INSTRUCTIONS

For Phase I of recovery from total knee replacement (up to 6 weeks postsurgery), do not add ankle weights.

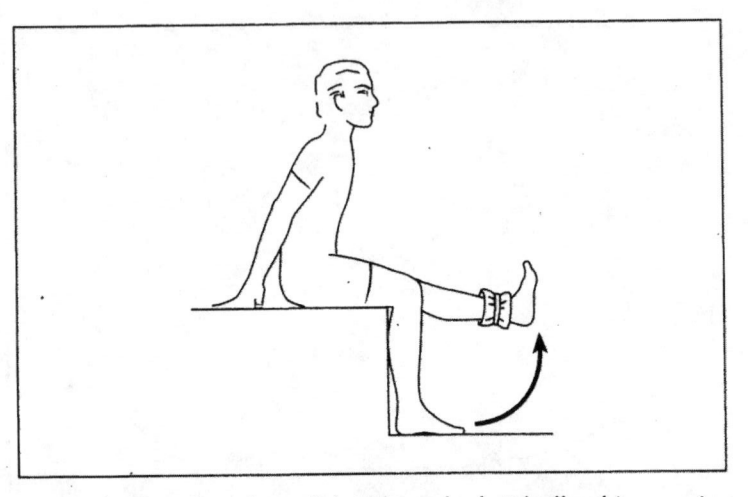

1. Sit on the edge of a solid table or bed. (Ideally, this exercise should be done without back support. However, if you need some support, you can sit on a straight-back chair.)
2. Extend your knee so that your leg is straight, but do not hyperextend. Raise and lower your leg from your knee. Raise your leg to a count of 4 and lower to a count of 8.
3. Repeat exercise 10 times. Do 2 more sets of 10.
4. As you get stronger, you can add 3- to 5-pound ankle weights to make the exercise more challenging.
5. Repeat exercise with other leg.

SPECIAL INSTRUCTIONS:

For ligament injuries, raise and lower your leg so that the foot actually touches the floor (which makes an arc of 90 degrees). This allows for full range of motion.

For patellar injuries, do not lower your leg more than halfway down (which makes an arc of 45 degrees).

If you have arthritis, lower your leg only about two-thirds of the way to the floor (which makes an arc of about 55 to 65 degrees).

For Phase I of recovery after total knee replacement (up to 6 weeks postsurgery), do not add ankle weights.

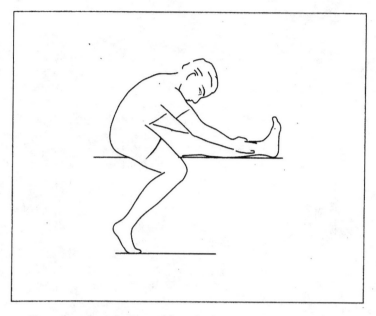

1. Sit on the edge of a firm table or bed.
2. Bend from the waist and slowly reach toward the toes of the extended leg. Hold the stretch for about 30 seconds. Stretch gently; *do not bounce.*
3. Repeat exercise 10 times. Do 2 more sets of 10.
4. Repeat exercise with other leg.

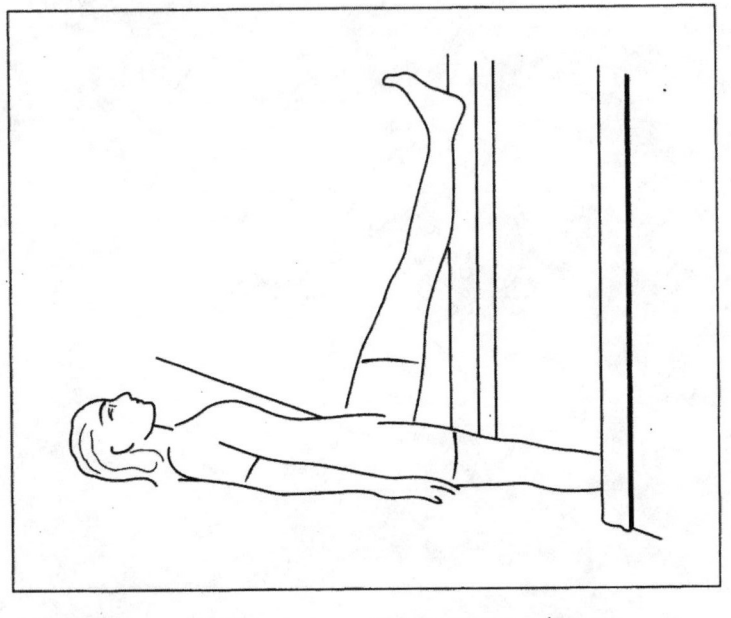

1. Lie down on the floor near a wall adjacent to a doorway.
2. Place one leg on the wall. Press that leg toward the wall with your foot and lower leg. Hold for about 30 seconds.
3. Slide your buttocks closer to the wall and repeat the exercise. Continue until your buttocks are as close to the wall as possible.
4. Repeat exercise 10 times. Do 2 more sets of 10.
5. Repeat exercise with other leg.

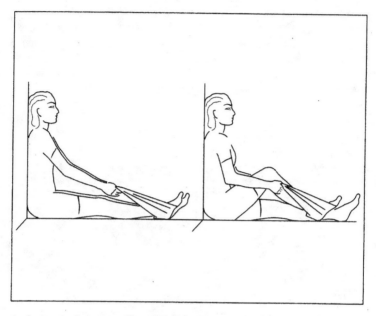

1. Lean against a wall with your back straight and your legs extended at a 90 degree angle to your back.
2. Wrap a rubber band (inexpensive exercise bands are sold at most sporting goods stores) around your foot at the ankle and then try to extend your knee against the resistance of the rubber band.
3. Hold for 30 seconds.
4. Repeat exercise 10 times. Do 2 more sets of 10.
5. Repeat exercise with other leg.

SPECIAL INSTRUCTIONS

For a ligament injury, flex your knee a full 90 degrees.

For arthritis, do not flex your knee more than 60 degrees.

For a patellar injury, do not flex your knee more than 40 degrees.

9 PRONE HIP EXTENSION

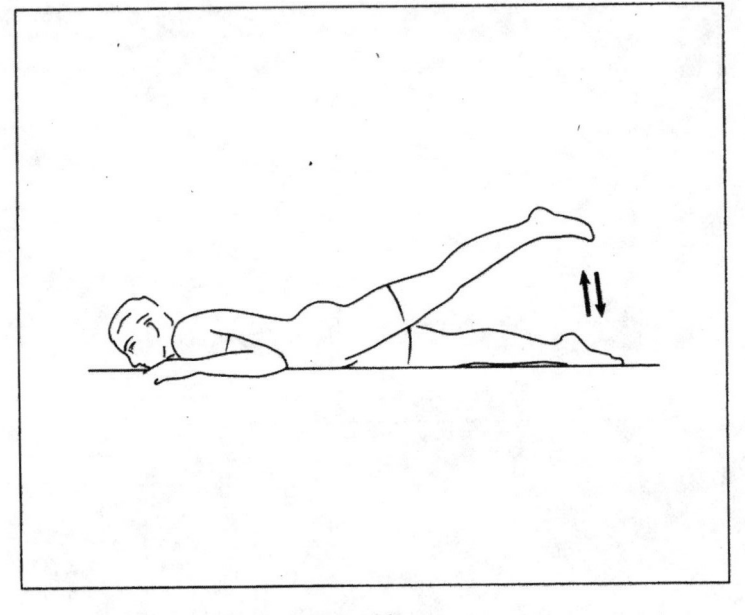

1. Lie face down on a flat, firm surface.
2. Raise your leg from the hip and slowly lower it. Raise your leg to a count of 4, and lower your leg to a count of 8.
3. Repeat exercise 10 times. Do 2 more sets of 10.
4. Repeat with other leg.

10a   PRONE RESISTED KNEE FLEXION

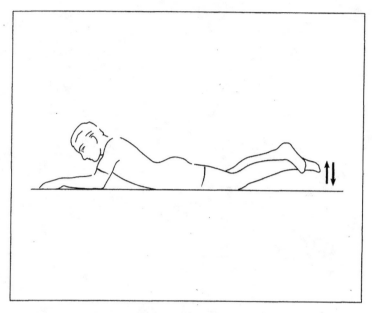

1. Lie face down on a flat, firm surface with legs straight. Place a pillow under your head for comfort.
2. Flex your knees to raise legs. Place the noninjured leg over the injured leg. (The injured leg is on the bottom.)
3. Push down with your noninjured leg while injured knee pushes up. Against resistance, bring legs back to floor.
4. Repeat exercise 10 times. Do 2 more sets of 10.

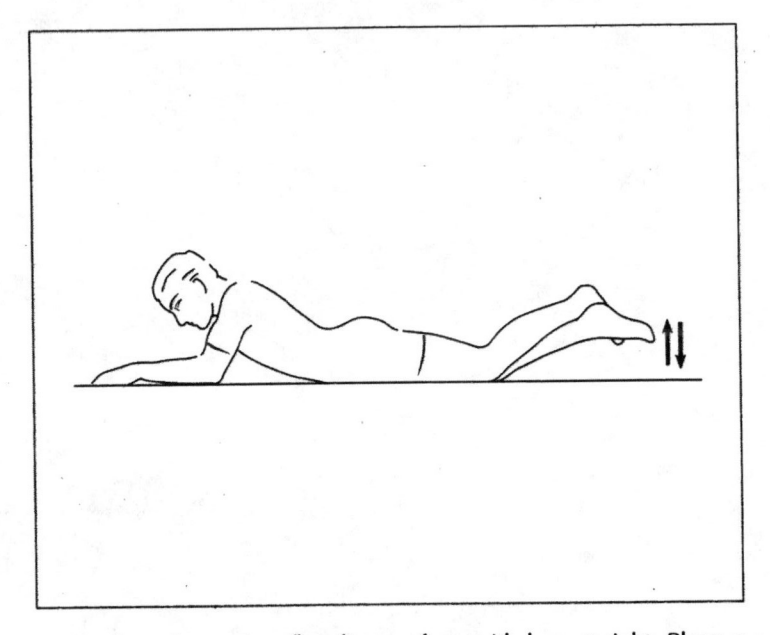

1. Lie face down on a flat, firm surface with legs straight. Place a pillow under your head for comfort.
2. Place the injured leg over the noninjured leg. (The noninjured leg is on the bottom.)
3. Push up with the bottom noninjured leg. The top leg is passive.
4. Repeat exercise 10 times. Do 2 more sets of 10.

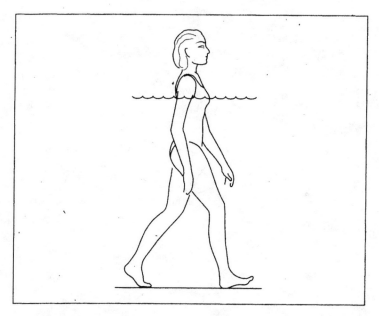

1. Walk briskly in chest-deep water. Start for 2 to 5 minutes, and gradually begin increasing your endurance until you can do this exercise for half an hour.

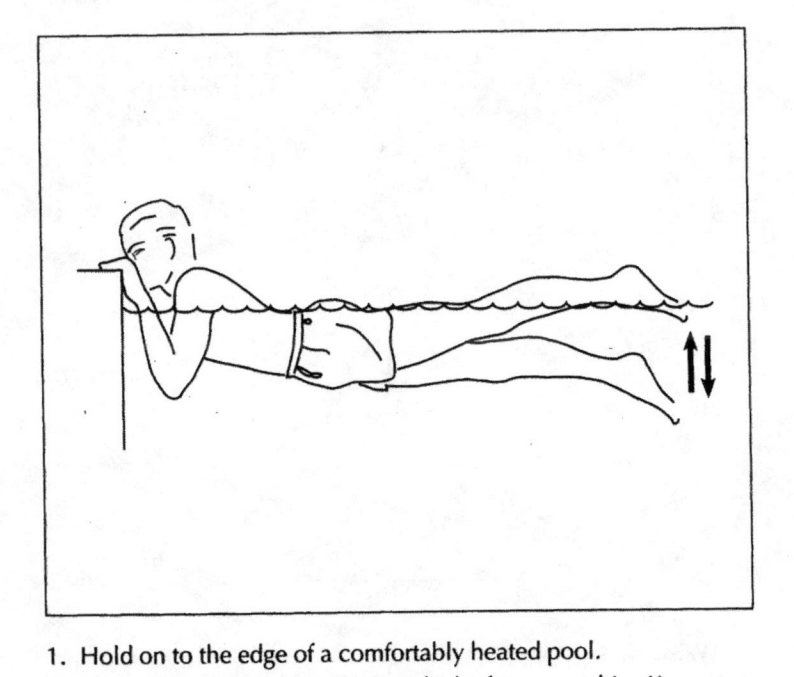

1. Hold on to the edge of a comfortably heated pool.
2. Extend legs and do small, short kicks from your hip. Keep your knees straight, but do not overextend them.
3. Start for 2 minutes, and gradually begin increasing your endurance until you can do this exercise for up to half an hour.

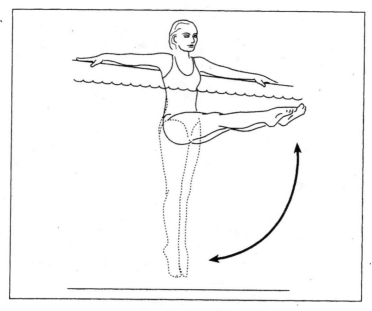

1. Stand with back against the side of the pool. Hold onto side.
2. Raise both legs to a 90 degree angle at the waist. Raise your legs to a count of 2, and lower them to a count of 4.
3. Repeat exercise 10 times. Do 2 more sets of 10.

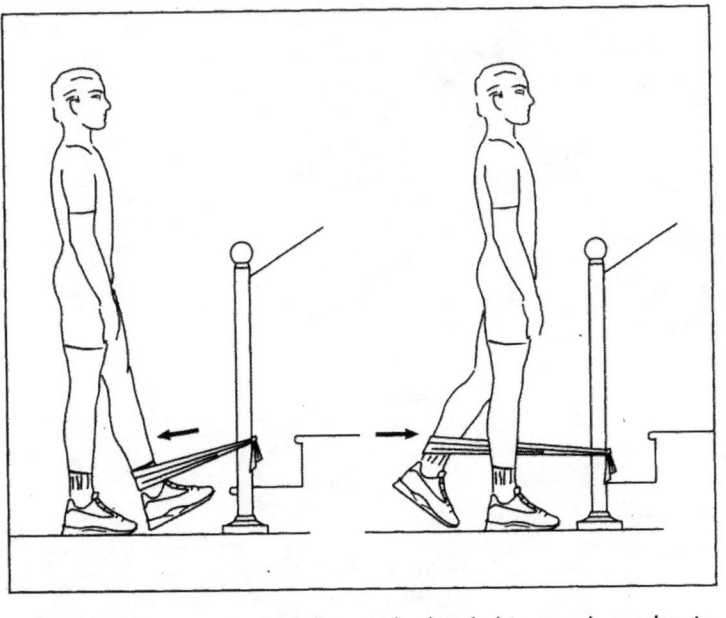

1. Tie a rubber exercise band around a fixed object such as a banister. (Inexpensive exercise bands are sold at most sporting goods stores.)
2. Wrap the band around your ankle. Extend and lower your leg from the hip against the resistance of the rubber band. Extend your leg to a count òf 4, and flex it to a count of 8.
3. Repeat exercise 10 times. Do 2 more sets of 10.
4. Repeat with other leg.

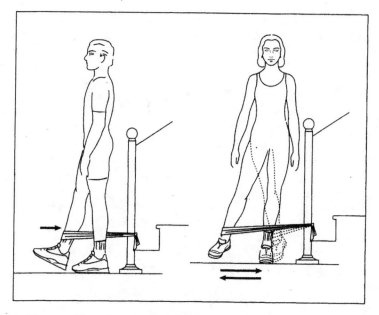

1. Tie a rubber exercise band around a fixed object such as a banister.
2. Wrap rubber band around ankle of one leg.
3. Flex the leg from the hip against the resistance of the rubber band. Extend your leg to a count of 4, and flex it to a count of 8.
4. Repeat exercise 10 times. Do 2 more sets of 10.

STANDING RUBBER BAND HIP ABDUCTION II

1. Secure a rubber exercise band around a fixed object such as a
   . banister.
2. Wrap the rubber band around your ankle.
3. Move your leg away from your hip, and pull against the resistance of the rubber band. Move your leg away to a count of 4, and return it to a count of 8.
4. Repeat exercise 10 times. Do 2 more sets of 10.

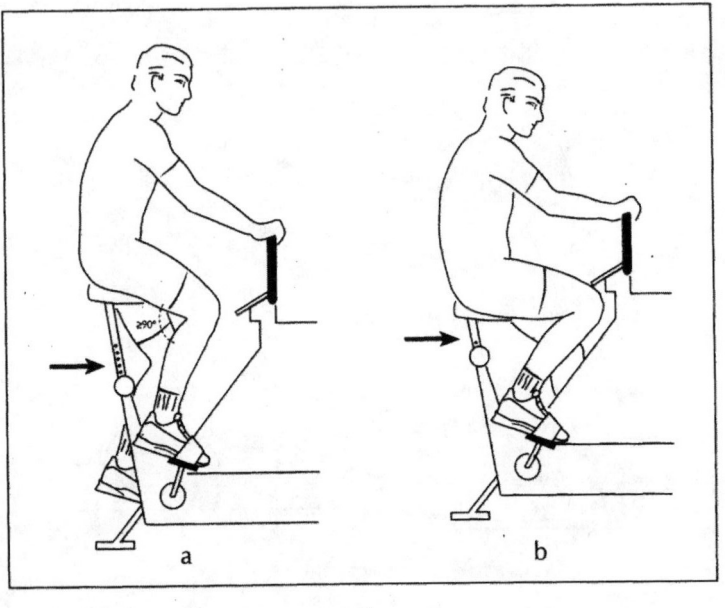

1. Secure your feet in the pedals.
2. Adjust the seat height according to your needs. If you have arthritis, a patellar injury, or a meniscal injury or have had a recent total knee replacement (within 6 weeks of surgery), make the seat high enough so that your knees are not bent more than 90 degrees (see A).

   If you have a ligament injury, lower the seat so that your knees are bent beyond 90 degrees to allow for a full range of motion. (see B).
3. Cycle for 15 minutes. As your endurance improves, you can cycle up to 30 to 40 minutes.
4. Do this exercise at least 3 times a week for maximum benefit.

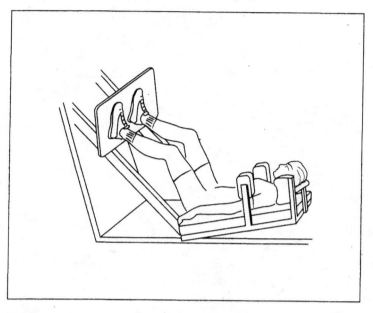

1. Lie down on the back cushion. Place both feet flat on the foot plate.
2. Using both legs, alternate between bending and extending the knees. The knees should not be bent more than 45 degrees.
3. Repeat exercise 10 times. Do 2 more sets of 10.

SPECIAL INSTRUCTIONS

For ligament injuries, flex your knees to 90 degrees.

For patellar injuries, do not flex your knees more than 45 degrees.

*To be done at rehabilitation center or gym.

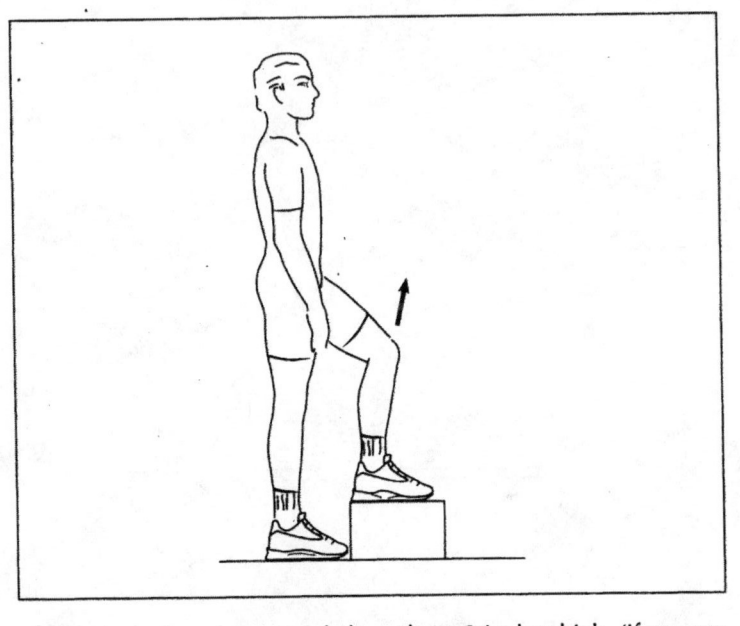

1. Place one leg onto a sturdy box about 8 inches high. (If you are under 5 feet, you may need to use a smaller box.)
2. Pull body up with lead leg. Try not to push off the floor with the rear leg. Your knee should not be bent more than 45 degrees.
3. Repeat exercise 10 times. Do 2 more sets of 10.
4. Change lead legs and repeat exercise.

SPECIAL INSTRUCTIONS

For a patellar injury, do not bend your knee more than 45 degrees.

Do not do this exercise if you are in pain.

During the recovery period after a total knee replacement, use a cane or railing to support your upper body.

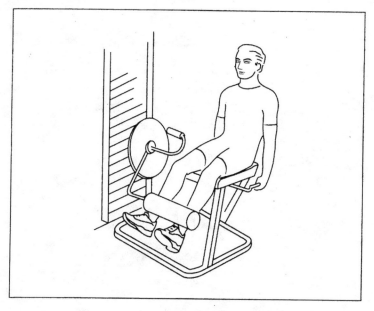

1. Sit straight in chair. Place hands on the support bar.
2. Alternate between raising the padded bar with your left and right legs. Slowly lower the bar. If this is too difficult, you can use both legs to raise the padded bar. Raise legs to count of 4, and lower them a count of 8.
3. Repeat exercise 10 times. Do 2 more sets of 10.

SPECIAL INSTRUCTIONS

Do not do this exercise if you are in pain.

If you have a patellar injury, do not bend your knee more than 45 degrees.

If you have had surgery for an anterior cruciate ligament injury, do not do this exercise until 5 to 6 weeks postsurgery.

*To be done at rehabilitation center or gym.

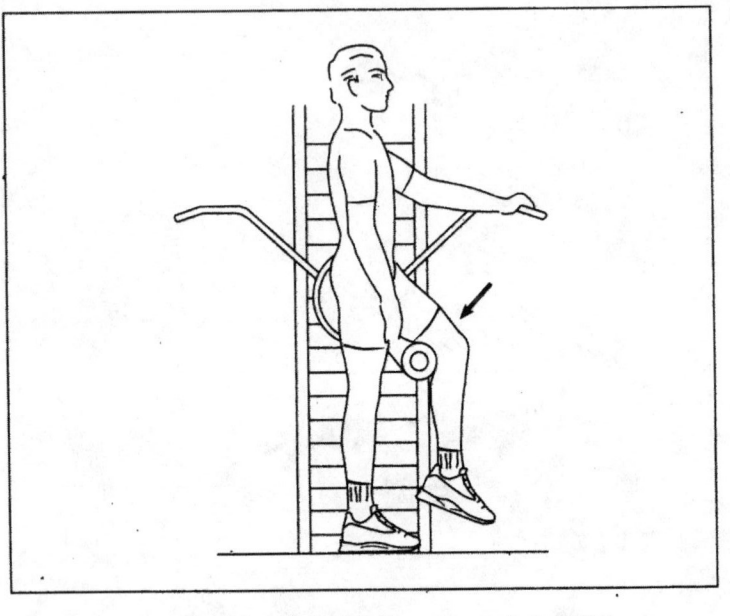

1. Place bolster pad behind and above your knee. Place arm on support bar. Push down with your upper thigh. Take 4 counts to push down and 8 counts to return to starting position.
2. Repeat exercise 10 times. Do 2 more sets of 10.

*To be done at rehabilitation center or gym.

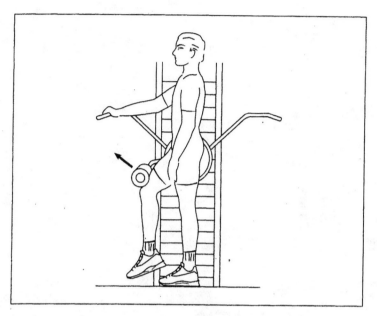

1. Place bolster pad in front of and above your knee. Place arm on support bar.
2. Push thigh upward to flex hip. Take 4 counts to push up and 8 counts to return to starting position.
3. Repeat exercise 10 times. Do 2 more sets of 10.

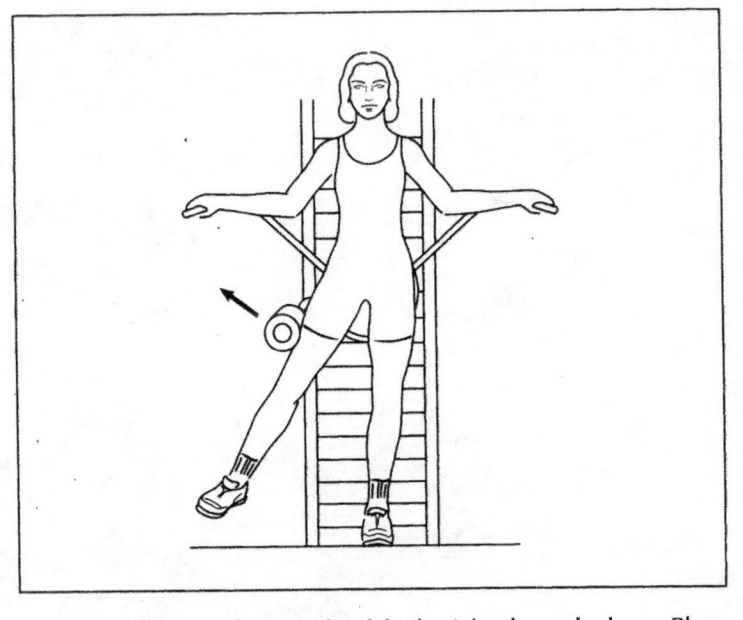

1. Place bolster on the outside of thigh, right above the knee. Place arms on support bars.
2. Push outward at hips. Take 4 counts to push out and 8 counts to return to starting position.
3. Repeat exercise 10 times. Do 2 more sets of 10.
4. Repeat exercise with other leg.

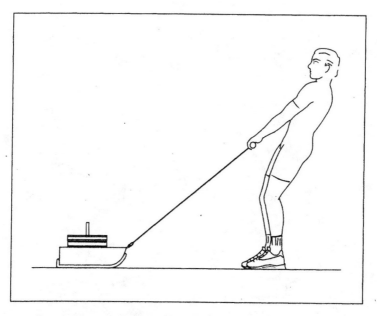

1. Fill a plastic milk crate with weights between one-third and two-thirds of your body weight. Use a hook to attach rope.
2. Holding onto the rope, drag the milk crate about 30 feet.
3. Repeat exercise 10 times. Do 2 more sets of 10.
4. When you can do three sets comfortably, increase the weight to make the exercise more challenging.

SPECIAL INSTRUCTIONS

If you have a cartilage injury (including a meniscal injury) or arthritis, stick with the lowest weights.

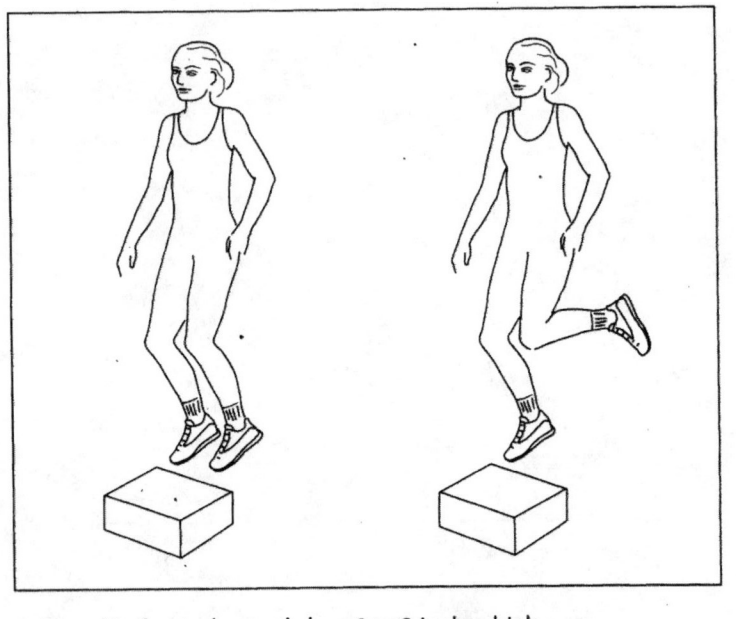

1. Stand in front of a sturdy box 6 to 8 inches high.
2. Jump on and off the box, alternating between single and double leg jumps.
3. Repeat exercise 10 times. Do 2 more sets of 10.

*This exercise is only for advanced patients and should not to be done by people who are in pain.

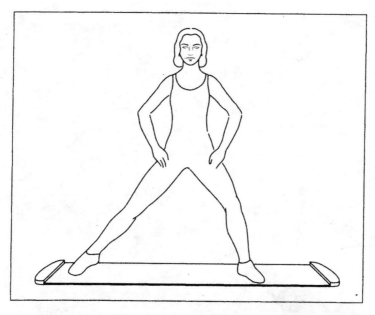

1. Stand on a 6- to 8-foot slide board. (Slide boards are sold at most sporting goods stores and on cable TV.) Wear wool socks or booties that are sold with slide board. While keeping your knees slightly bent, glide from left to right across the board.
2. Begin by trying to slide back and forth for 30 seconds. Keep increasing your time on the slide board until you can stay on up to 5 to 10 minutes.

SPECIAL INSTRUCTIONS

If you have had surgery for an injured ligament, do not do this exercise until six weeks postsurgery.

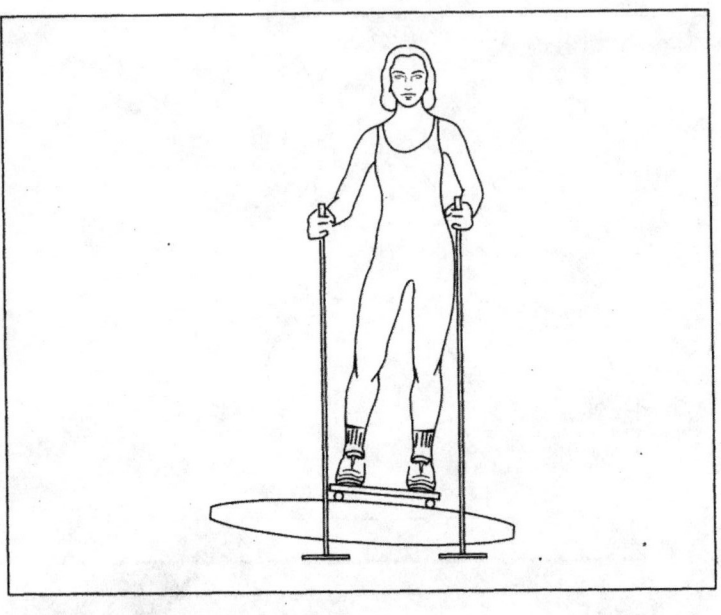

1. Place a roller board on an arched surface. (Both pieces of equipment can be purchased at most exercise or sporting goods stores.) Stand on the roller board (which is on the platform) and shift your body weight from left to right. Ski poles can be used to mimic the skiing motion.
2. Begin by trying to stay on board for 2 minutes. As you become more proficient at maintaining your balance, you can work your way up to 10 minutes.

SPECIAL INSTRUCTIONS

If you have had surgery for an injured ligament, do not do this exercise until 6 weeks postsurgery.

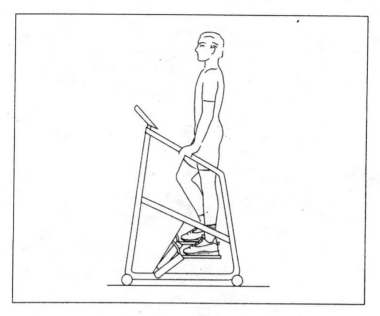

1. Set machine for *low* resistance. Using *short steps only,* walk briskly on the pedals. You can hold the side rails for support if necessary.
2. Begin by staying on the stair climber for 5 to 10 minutes, and gradually work up to 30 minutes.

*Stair climbers should not be used at high resistance because they can damage knees, and should not be used by anyone with patellar pain.

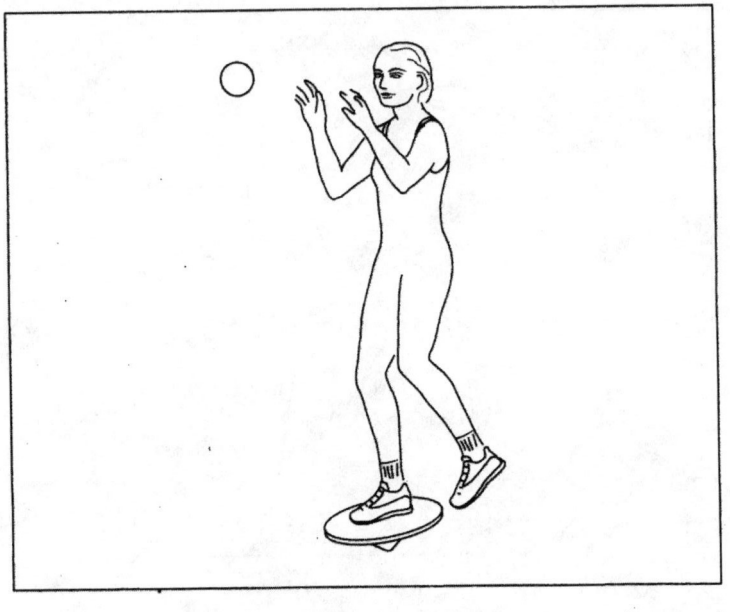

1. While balancing on a balance board, alternate catching and throwing balls of different weights. (Balance boards can be purchased at most sporting goods stores.)

*This exercise is for advanced patients only and should not be done by people who are still in pain.

INDEX

Printed in the United States
By Bookmasters